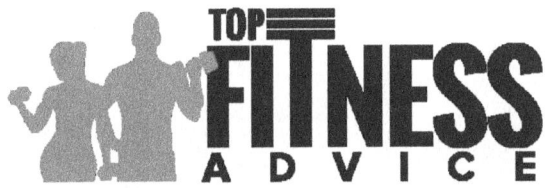

THE FASTEST WAY TO LOSE WEIGHT

A Beginner's Guide To HIIT For Faster Weight Loss

Sarah Talene

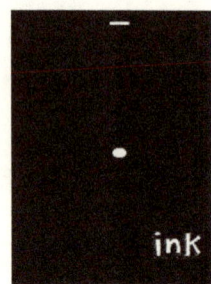

First published in 2017 by Venture Ink Publishing

Copyright © Top Fitness Advice 2019

All rights reserved.

No part of this book may be reproduced in any form without permission in writing from the author. No part of this publication may be reproduced or transmitted in any form or by any means, mechanic, electronic, photocopying, recording, by any storage or retrieval system, or transmitted by email without the permission in writing from the author and publisher.

Requests to the publisher for permission should be addressed to
publishing@ventureink.co

For more information about the contents of this book or questions to the author, please contact Sarah Talene at
sarah@topfitnessadvice.com

Disclaimer

This book provides wellness management information in an informative and educational manner only, with information that is general in nature and that is not specific to you, the reader. The contents of this book are intended to assist you and other readers in your personal wellness efforts. Consult your physician regarding the applicability of any information provided in this book to you.

Nothing in this book should be construed as personal advice or diagnosis, and must not be used in this manner. The information provided about conditions is general in nature. This information does not cover all possible uses, actions, precautions, side-effects, or interactions of medicines, or medical procedures. The information in this book should not be considered as complete and does not cover all diseases, ailments, physical conditions, or their treatment.

You should consult with your physician before beginning any exercise, weight loss, or health care program. This book should not be used in place of a call or visit to a competent health-care professional. You should consult a health care professional before adopting any of the suggestions in this book or before drawing inferences from it.

Any decision regarding treatment and medication for your condition should be made with the advice and consultation of a qualified health care professional. If you have, or suspect you have, a health-care problem, then you should immediately contact a qualified health care professional for treatment.

No Warranties: The author and publisher don't guarantee or warrant the quality, accuracy, completeness, timeliness, appropriateness or suitability of the information in this book, or of any product or services referenced in this book.

The information in this book is provided on an "as is" basis and the author and publisher make no representations or warranties of any kind with respect to this information. This book may contain inaccuracies, typographical errors, or other errors.

Liability Disclaimer: The publisher, author, and other parties involved in the creation, production, provision of information, or delivery of this book specifically disclaim any responsibility, and shall not be held liable for any damages, claims, injuries, losses, liabilities, costs, or obligations including any direct, indirect, special, incidental, or consequences damages (collectively known as "Damages") whatsoever and howsoever caused, arising out of, or in connection with the use or misuse of the site and the information contained within it, whether such Damages arise in contract, tort, negligence, equity, statute law, or by way of other legal theory.

Table of Contents

Disclaimer	3
Who is this book for?	7
What will this book teach you?	9
Introduction	11
Chapter 1: Understanding How HIIT Works	17
Chapter 2: Assessing Your Level of Fitness Now	21
Chapter 3: Structuring Your Workouts	25
Chapter 4: Workouts That Blast Fat	38
Chapter 5: The Main Reason You Can't Lose Weight	93
Chapter 6: Your Fat Blasting Food Plan	101
Chapter 7: Keeping It Up	109
Conclusion	117
Final Words	119

Would you prefer to listen to my book, rather than read it?

Download the audiobook version for free!

If you go to the special link below and sign up to Audible as a new customer, you can get the audiobook version of my book completely free.

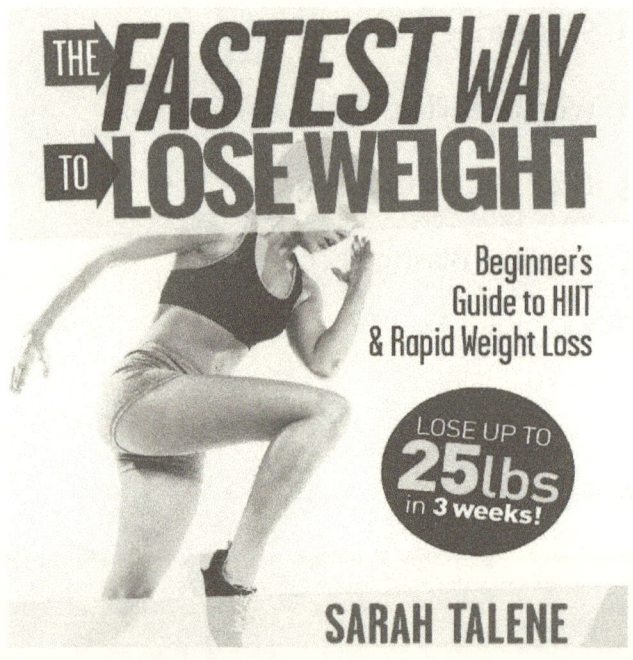

Go here to get your audiobook version for free:

TopFitnessAdvice.com/go/hiit

Who is this book for?

Are you sick of trying the latest crash diet, losing weight and then having it all pile back on again?

Do you feel like you will never lose the extra weight, no matter how hard you try?

If you are anything like I was, you would have tried every diet, diet pill and expensive gadget that ever came onto the market.

And, if you're honest, the only thing you have to show for all that effort and expense is a waistline that is bigger than it was before and a bunch of obsolete equipment in the garage.

Stop wasting your time and money now.

This book is going to turn what you think you know about diet and exercise on its head.

If you want faster, better and longer-lasting results, this is the book for you.

What will this book teach you?

The book is laid out in easy to follow sections.

I go through the basics of HIIT explaining about the RPE Scale so that you learn how to measure your overall level of exertion. We also look at why HIIT is so much more effective. We look at whether it is better to extend your workout at a lower rate or focus on a shorter, higher intensity workout.

In the second chapter, I have laid out a number of fitness tests that you can perform on yourself now to gauge your current level of fitness.

We go through what tools you might need to get the most out of your workouts and we talk about proper safety procedures.

After going through the full Warmup Routine, we head straight on to the exercise program.

The exercises can be done as and when you have time. Choose a five-minute workout for those days when you are rushing or choose a workout that focuses on your particular problem areas.

We do spend some time in the book going through what you should and should not eat. I have included a sample seven day eating plan to get you started.

Finally, we go through ways to maintain your motivation levels.

Introduction

I have been in the fitness industry for a number of years now. Fads come and go – we are all looking for the quick fix when it comes to health and weight loss.

Most of the time, the fads lose popularity quickly because they are too hard to maintain, too boring or too difficult.

I remember not wanting to ever eat cabbage again after following the Cabbage Soup Diet for a few days.

Fads come and go in much the same way when it comes to exercise as well. And that usually means buying expensive equipment or DVDs that end up cluttering up a corner of the garage.

It's time to give up on the fads. The only way that you are going to get the body of your dreams and be able to maintain it is if you are willing to put some effort in.

And here's the great news – your body is designed to move. It wants to be fit and healthy. And your body is the only piece of specialized equipment that you really need.

With the program laid out in this book, you are going to start seeing incredible results in a manner of weeks. The program in this book gives you measurable results fast, just like a fad diet would. The difference here is that these results are sustainable.

The program is centered on High Intensity Interval Training (HIIT). HIIT has been scientifically proven to be extremely effective when it comes to reshaping your body. It is so effective, in fact, that you get to spend less time exercising and get better results.

In this book, I will teach you how the workouts work, which workouts to do, how to measure progress and how to get the best possible results.

I will also give you an introduction into cleaning up your dietary habits and a sample week-long program for you to follow.

If you are tired of programs that overpromise and underdeliver, HIIT is the answer. Kick out the fads that don't work and start working out at a whole new level.

Weight Loss is HARD!

Discover How to Make It EASIER to Lose Weight & Keep It OFF Forever (This Is The ONLY Book You NEED to Read)

For this month only, you can get Sarah's best-selling & most popular guide absolutely free – *The #1 Weight Loss Guide*.

Get Your FREE Copy Here:

TopFitnessAdvice.com/Freebie

It's time to stop struggling with your weight loss efforts that don't seem to work.

Discover how you can start seeing real results by next week (without changing much in your life). With this guide, readers were able to significantly improve their weight loss results. So, it's highly recommended that you get this guide, especially while it's free!

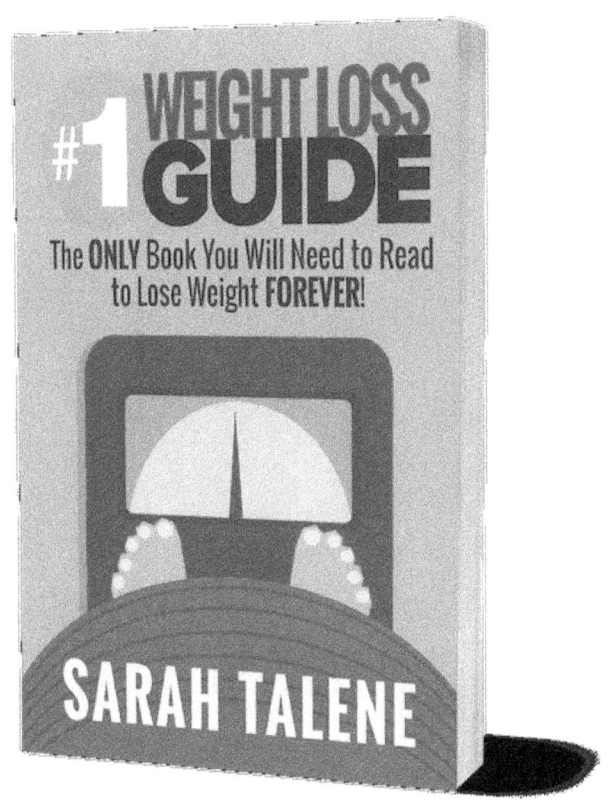

Get Your FREE Copy Here:

TopFitnessAdvice.com/Freebie

Chapter 1

Understanding How HIIT Works

You may have heard of intermittent or interval training already. These are both other ways to describe HIIT.

What makes HIIT really stand out is that it can be used in conjunction with any fitness program that you like. It can be applied to walking or running, swimming, etc. You get to see results in a much shorter period of time and this helps you to maintain your motivation levels.

Throughout the course of this book, we will be referring to the intensity of the exercise or the RPE rating.

The RPE Scale

As the intensity of the exercise is what is important here, we need to adopt a slightly different scale of measurements.

The RPE Scale is ideal because it allows you to determine how much you are exerting yourself.

The scale runs from 1 – 10. 1 on the scale means that you are not exerting yourself at all. 10 on the scale means that you are exerting yourself as much as you are able.

By assigning a numerical value to the level of exertion in this way, you can ensure that you are working hard enough to make a difference.

For the most part in this training, we will not exceed level 7. Most exercises will start at level 4. Occasionally we might increase the exertion to level 8.

It is not wise to exceed level 8 as you will then be putting too much stress on your body. Your body goes into survival mode and, instead of burning fat, holds onto its stores for as long as it is able to.

Rev Up Your Fat Burning

Interval training is particularly effective for cranking up the fat burning ability of your body.

Research has shown that it is more important to train at different levels of exertion than to stick to just one level over a longer period. It is believed that exercising at just one level of exertion makes it easier for the body to become used to the exercise.

Once it knows what is coming, the body will be able to perform the actions in the most energy efficient way. Interval training means that the body is always kept guessing.

In addition, these intense bursts of exercise can help you tone and shape up like nothing else does.

Interval training reduces the time needed to shape the body and reduces the recovery time needed as well.

And you aren't just benefiting while at the gym. Your body continues to burn fat at an increased rate for hours after you have finished exercising.

And, better still, you can slot HIIT training into your daily life. Grab five minutes during your lunch hour and you can fit in a mini-workout.

If you are looking for an exercise plan to end all excuses, this is it. There is no such thing as, "I don't have the time to exercise" or "I just couldn't make it to the gym." Excuses are a thing of the past now.

Higher Intensity or Longer Duration?

Research has shown that it is the intensity at which we exercise rather than the total amount of exercise that makes the difference.
It has been proven that you will get the same benefits from three separate 10 minute sessions of exercise that you will if you did it all in one block.

Increasing the intensity of the workouts make them even more effective so you are able to get better results without needing to spend extra time exercising.

What this means for you is that the 7-minute workout that you do at high intensity does you a lot more good than a more gentle half an hour workout would do.

High Intensity improves the health of your cardiovascular system, helps to reduce stress, increases the amount of fat your body burns, helps to tone, reduces the time needed to recover, improves your health overall and helps you to feel a lot better. And it does all of this in a lot less time than a standard workout would.

Chapter 2

Assessing Your Level of Fitness Now

You do need to know what your current level of fitness is and this chapter is going to help you measure that.

The tests in this chapter can be repeated at regular intervals so that you can see how you are progressing. I recommend doing the tests every three months or so.

The Tests

In the tests, you simply need to record either how long it took you to complete the task or how many repetitions you were able to complete in the allotted time.

The Mile-Long Test

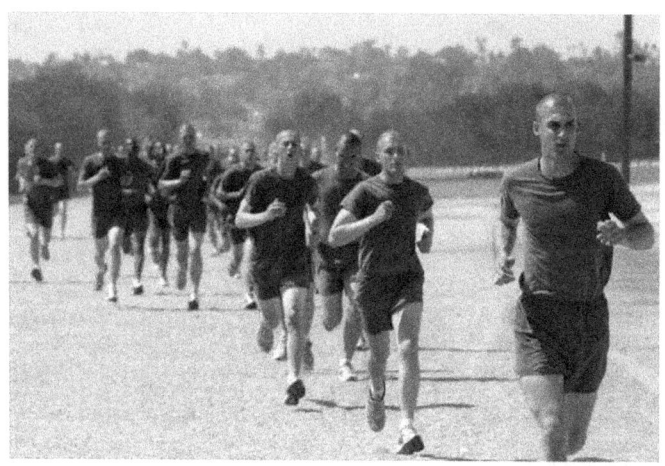

This is a very simple one. Measure out a route of one mile. Now either walk or run that mile, timing yourself. You want to complete it as quickly as you are able.

If you have not done much exercise in the last few years, it is better to walk this distance rather than trying to run it.

Make a note of the date of the test, how long it took you and how you felt it went. (Was it easy, etc?)

Push-Ups

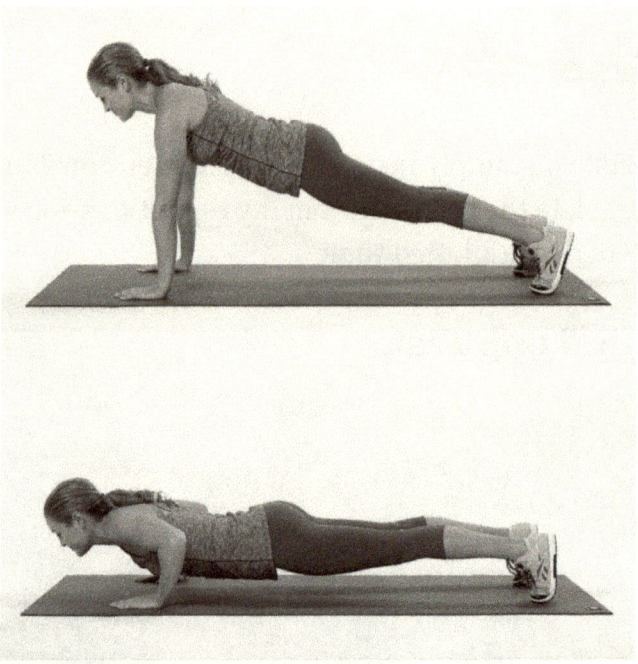

These will help test your upper-body strength. If you haven't exercised much recently, start by doing push-ups from the knee instead of full pushups.

For this exercise, just do as many pushups as you can manage before you are too tired to continue.

Alternatively, set the timer for 3-5 minutes and do as many as you can manage during that time.

Make a note of how many you could do and how you felt it went.

Walking Lunges

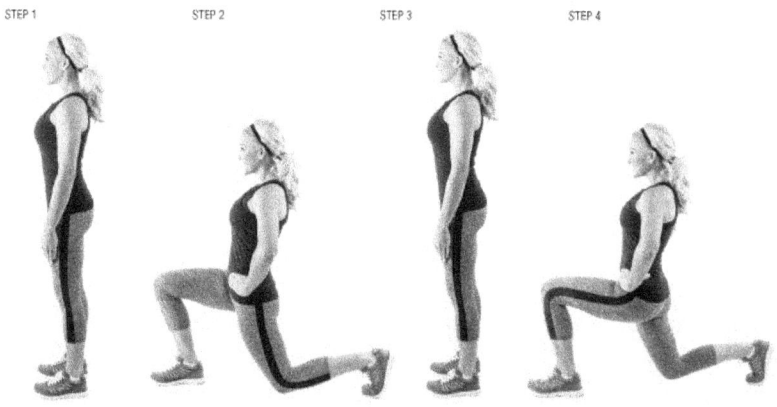

These will help you test your lower-body strength. Again, all you need to do is to do lunges until you are too tired to do any more.

You can also set your timer and see how many you are able to complete in the allotted time frame.

How Well You Feel

This test has no real objective measurements. You simply write down how you are feeling on a scale from one to ten. The better you feel, the higher the score you can assign yourself.

The further along you get in this program, the better you will feel overall.

Measurements

The scale is one way of seeing whether or not you are making progress when it comes to losing weight. Unfortunately, it is not the most accurate measure.

Your weight can fluctuate on a daily basis, making results achieved this way less reliable.

If you want a more accurate record of your progress, a tape measure is a much better ally.

Measure your waist at its narrowest point.

Measure your upper thigh at its widest point.

Measure your hips at their widest point.

Measure your upper arms at their widest point.

When doing follow-up measurements, be sure to measure in the same place again.

I hope that you are enjoying this book so far, and if you could spare 30 seconds, I would greatly appreciate you leaving a review on Amazon.com.

Chapter 3

Structuring Your Workouts

Most of the exercises in this book can easily be done at home with minimal equipment. There are some things that I do recommend that you do get.

Your Shoes

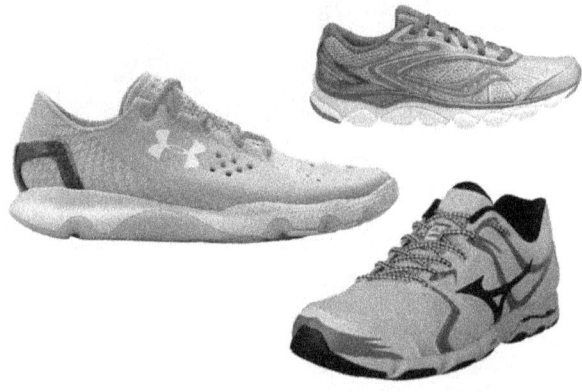

You need a good pair of shoes to work out in. This is especially important when you are doing high-impact exercises. It is worth spending a bit more on these shoes so that you get a better level of protection.

If your shoes are well-worn and no longer providing the support that they should, they need to be replaced.

Shoes that fit badly, shoes that have seen better days or shoes that offer no support at all could increase your chances of injuring yourself.

For the Ladies

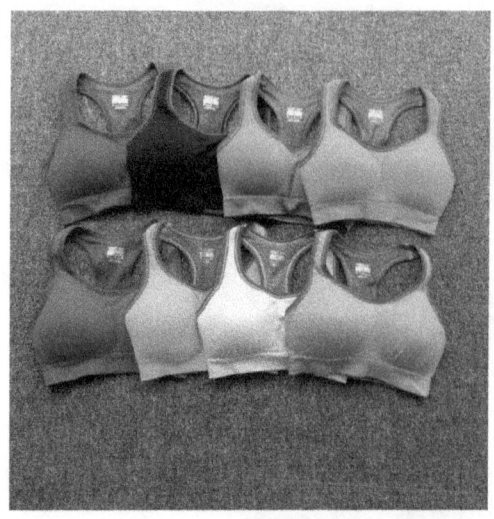

Ladies need to ensure that they are wearing a proper sports bra. Exercise can be hard on the breasts because of the increased movement. The last thing that you want is for your breasts to jiggle all over the place.

A Timer

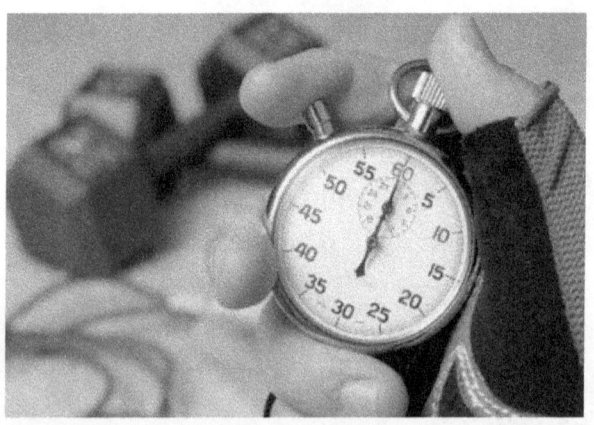

You can either buy a timer or use the one on your phone. If you don't find one on your phone, download one of the many apps available for this.

A stopwatch can be a good investment. They do not cost much and so it might be worth getting one just for workouts.

For the Floor

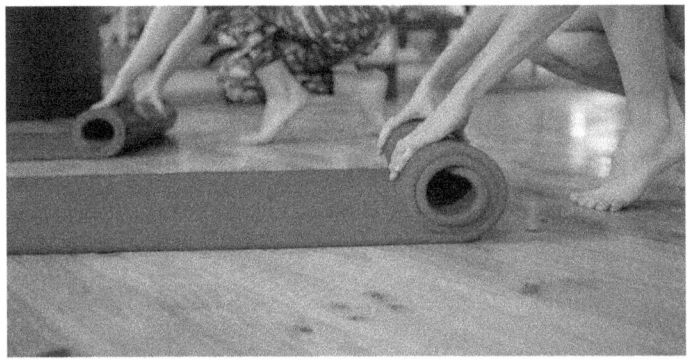

It is a good idea to have a floor mat or large towel for when you are doing floor exercises.

Weights

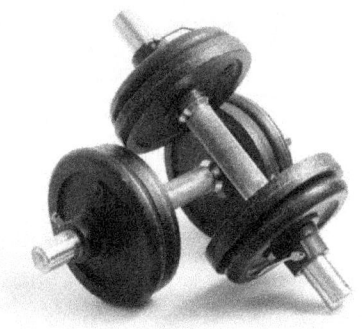

A good set of free weights will be with you for a long time and will always be useful. If you like, you can use cans of food or bottles of water, etc. as makeshift weights. I do advise that you get a set of weights as soon as you are able.

Jumping Rope

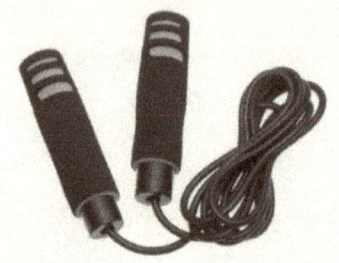

Jumping ropes are one of the best exercise tools you can own. They don't cost much so do get yourself one.

Allocate an Area

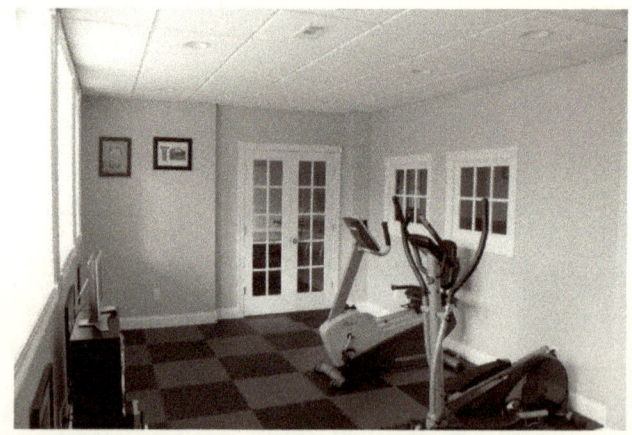

Set aside an area that you can exercise in. Place all your exercise equipment there so that you have it on hand as you need it. If the equipment is packed away, you are more likely to make excuses about not getting it out.

Clothing

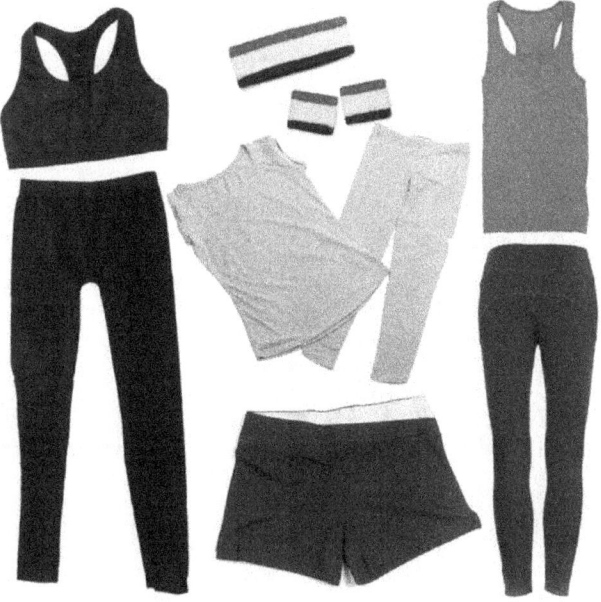

You do not have to go out and spend a fortune on clothes for gym. Make sure that you choose clothes that are comfortable to work out in. Natural fibers breathe better during workouts.

If you do plan to exercise on the streets, make sure that your clothing makes you highly visible to motorists.

Reaching the Right Intensity to Workout At

RPE Scale	Rate of Perceived Exertion
10	**Max Effort Activity** Feels almost impossible to keep going. Completely out of breath, unable to talk. Cannot maintain for more than a very short time.
9	**Very Hard Activity** Very difficult to maintain exercise intensity. Can barely breath and speak only a few words
7-8	**Vigorous Activity** Borderline uncomfortable. Short of breath, can speak a sentence.
4-6	**Moderate Activity** Breathing heavily, can hold short conversation. Still somewhat comfortable, but becoming noticeably more challenging.
2-3	**Light Activity** Feels like you can maintain for hours. Easy to breathe and carry a conversation
1	**Very Light Activity** Hardly any exertion, but more than sleeping, watching TV, etc

You are going to use the RPE scale to determine what the ideal workout level for you is. As everyone is at different levels of fitness, it is far better to rely on this scale than to insist on a set number of sets, etc.

Here is what each number on the scale represents:

1 – No exertion
2 – A very small amount of exertion (Getting up to go somewhere)
3 - Very light exertion (Gently exercising)
4 - Moderate exertion
5 - Somewhat hard exertion (Still able to hold a conversation)

6 - Hard (No long able to hold a conversation)
7 - Very hard
8 - Very, very hard
9 - Near exhaustion
10 - Maximum

Warming-Up and Cooling Down

Stretching is a low-intensity exercise so it can be skipped if you are short on time, can't it?

Always take the time to stretch your body before working out.

This helps to warm the muscles before you get into the actual exercise and reduces the chance of injuring yourself during the exercises.

Your muscles need to be eased into exercise, at least at first. When they are cold, the stiffen up and this reduces the amount that you can move them.

If you want the best workout possible, you have to stretch first.

It is also advisable to march in place for about a minute or two when you are finished working out to allow your body to come back to normal again.

Your Warm-Up Routine

You can start off by simply walking in place for a minute or two. Once you have done this, add another minute where you lift your legs higher. At the same time, raise your arms to shoulder height and move them in a large circular motion.

If you have access to stairs, walking up and down them a few times can be helpful.

The following exercises will help to complete your warm-up routine. You can also do this set of exercises at the end of your workout so that the muscles are stretched and smoothed back into place.

Calf Stretch

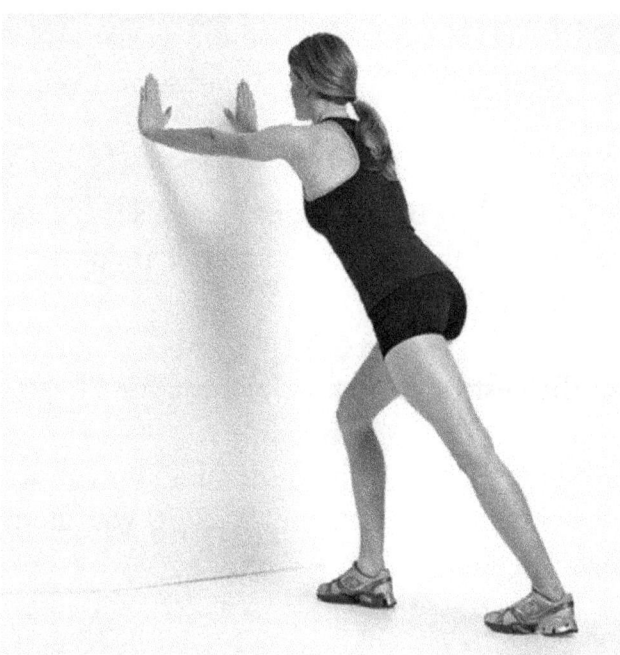

Take a step back with your right leg. Keep your right leg straight and bend your left leg at the knee. Feel the stretch in the right leg. Hold it for 10 seconds. Repeat on the other side.

Hamstring Stretch

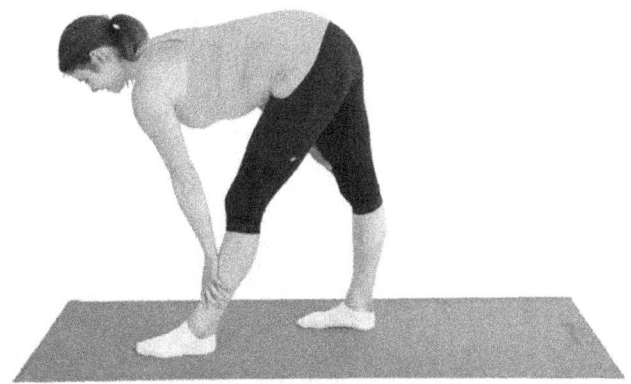

Step forward using your right leg. Keeping the heel of the right foot on the floor, bend at the knee. Reach down and hold the left leg. The stretch should be felt at the back of your left leg. Hold it for 10 seconds. Repeat on the other side.

Quadriceps Stretch

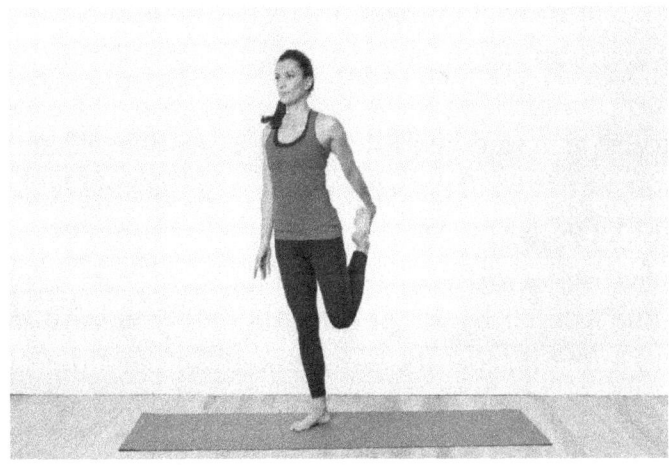

Be sure that you are standing up straight. Bend your left leg at the knee and raise the left foot so that it meets your buttock. Keep the right knee loose and slightly bent.

Hold it for 10 seconds. Repeat on the other side.

Triceps Stretch

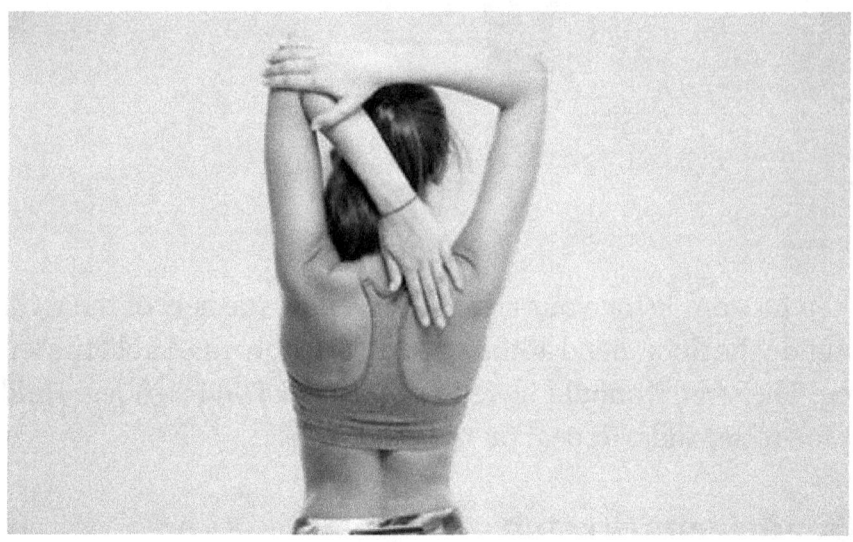

Be sure that you are standing up straight. Bend the knees a little and pull your tummy in.

Lift your left arm and bend it at the elbow. Reach behind your head with your hand. Try to get as close to the area between the shoulder blades as you can.

Deepen the stretch by supporting the left arm with the right one. Hold it for 10 seconds. Repeat on the other side.

Chest Stretch

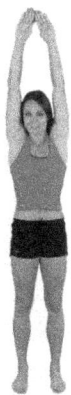

Be sure to stand up straight and stretch your arms up above your head. You should feel the stretch in the shoulders, chest and back.

Hold it for 10 seconds. Repeat on the other side.

Back Stretch

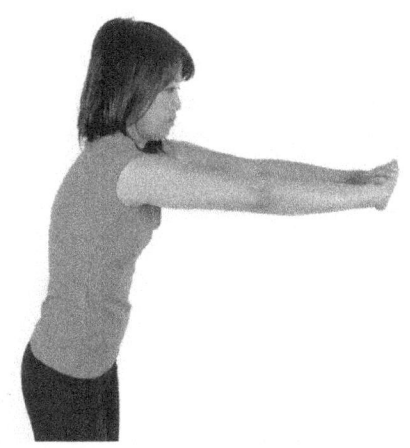

Be sure to stand up straight. Make sure that the knees are not locked and that your tummy is pulled in completely. Hold your arms straight out ahead of you and imagine that you are cuddling a teddy. You will feel the stretch in the back and the back of the arms.

Hold it for 10 seconds. Repeat on the other side.

Keeping Safe

We won't try and rush through things because we believe that this will pay dividends at the end of the day.

If you feel as though you are just going to rush through a workout, it is better to shelve it or you could do yourself more harm than good.

- Always leave time to warm-up before exercising and cool down after exercising. Injuries will set you back even more.

- Be sure to take heed of what your body is telling you. A little bit of discomfort in the beginning is perfectly natural, especially if you haven't exercised in a while. Don't push past the pain if it becomes too much. If you have hurt yourself, stop for the day.

- Always drink enough water.

- When exercising outside, be sure to wear clothes that are highly visible.

- If you are feeling sickly, it is best not to work out

If You Do Get Hurt

If you do injure yourself whilst exercising, you should stop there and then.

If you have inflammation or swelling, apply an icepack to the area and rest it for a while. Do not leave the icepack on for longer than twenty minutes.

If you find that the injury is still extremely sore, despite the icepack or if you are unable to walk, it is best to see a doctor as soon as possible.

Once again, thank you for reading this book, and I hope you're getting a lot of valuable information. I would greatly appreciate it if you could take 30 seconds to leave me a review for this book on Amazon.com.

Chapter 4

Workouts That Blast Fat

Now that we have covered the basics, let's get down to the workouts. With all these exercises, you need to do the warm-up as listed in the previous chapter before you start. Do the same exercises again to cool down after exercising.

The 4-Minute Fat Blast

Tones: The arms, abs, bottom and thighs
RPE: 5 to 7

This is a timed exercise so get out your stopwatch.
This is an extremely simple exercise to do. You will alternate the fat burning workout with walking in place.

Part 1: Deep Squat Star

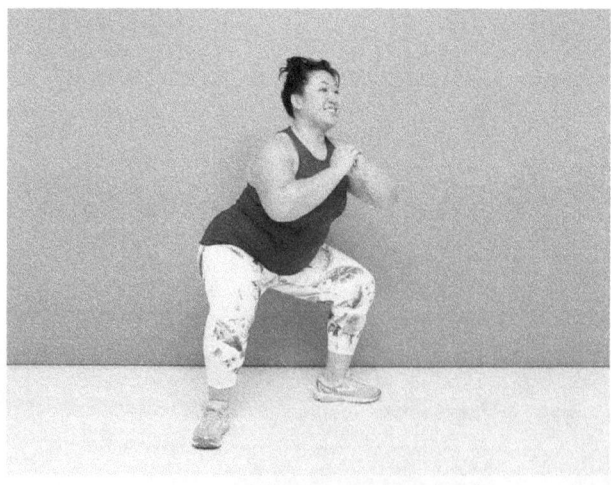

1. Position yourself in a deep squat. Hold this position for a few second and then jump up as high as you are able.

2. Throw your arms up in the air and spread the legs wide.

3. Return to the original position when the jump is over. Do this exercise as many times as you can for 20 seconds.

4. March in place for 10 seconds. This can be a slow march to help you recover.

Part 2: Knees Up

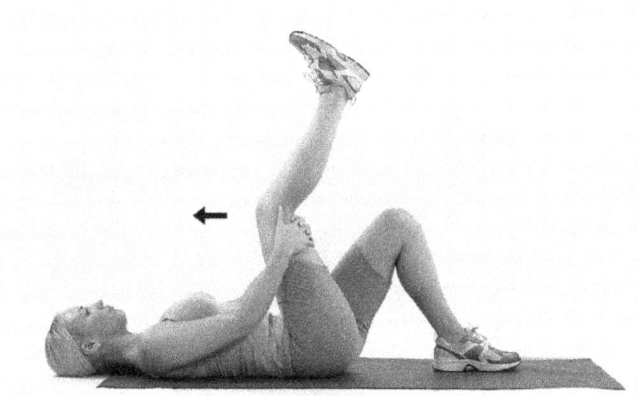

1. Lower yourself to the floor on your back.

2. Put your hands a little ahead of where your shoulders are and bring your left knee up to your chest.

3. Hold the knee in place for a second or two. Repeat on the other side. Do this exercise as many times as you can for 20 seconds.

4. March in place for 10 seconds. Repeat the whole sequence three times over.

The 5-Minute Fat Blaster

Tones: The arms, legs, bottom, thighs, abs, and waist.
RPE: 5 to 7

Part 1: The Skater's Lunge

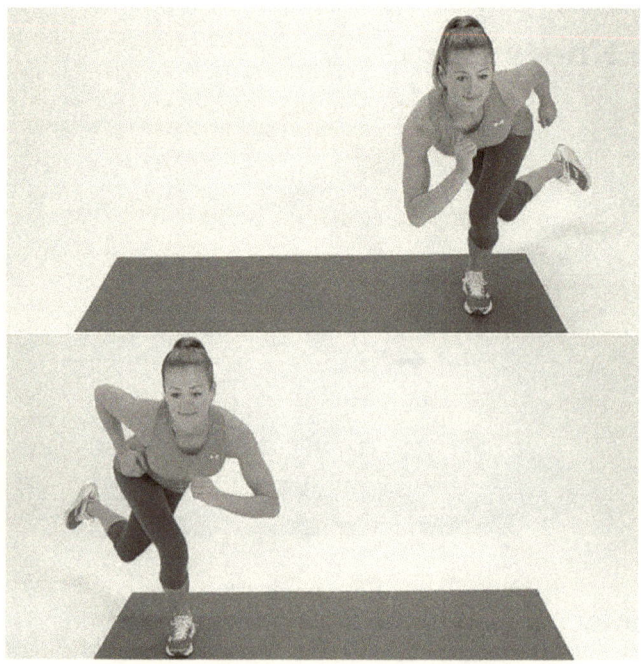

1. Step back with your right foot so that it is behind you diagonally and your heel is lifted.

2. Lower yourself into a lunge, ensuring that your left knee stays behind the toe line.

3. Raise your left arm so that it is out and to the side. Bring the right arm across to meet it.

4. Jump, switching the position of both the arms and the legs. Repeat on each side for a total of 50 seconds.

5. Rest by walking in place slowly for 10 seconds.

Part 2: Rope Pull for the Abdominals

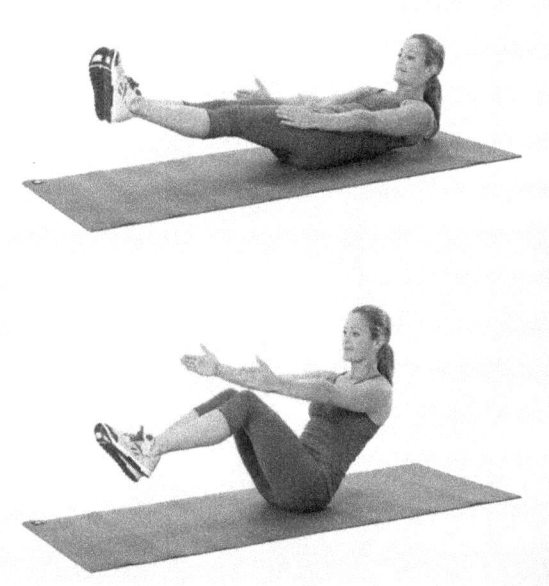

1. Lower yourself to the floor onto your back. Imagine that there is a length of rope coiled around your feet and that one end is in your hands.

2. Climb this "rope" using your arms. At the same time, lift your legs as if they were being pulled by the rope.

3. Climb as high as you are able. Do this exercise as many times as you can in 50 seconds.

4. Rest by walking in place for 10 seconds.

Part 3: Cannonball Squat

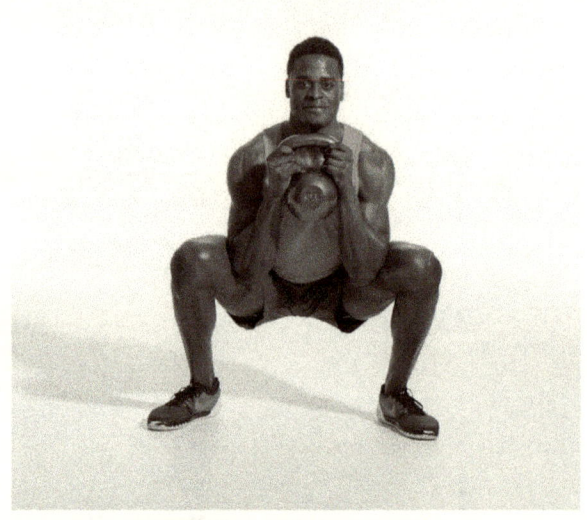

1. Lower yourself into a deep squat.

2. Do three deep squats, all the while ensuring that your knees stay behind your toes.

3. Jump as high as you can from this position, returning to it as you land. Do this exercise as many times as you can in 50 seconds.

4. Rest by walking in place for 10 seconds.

Part 4: Plank Lunge

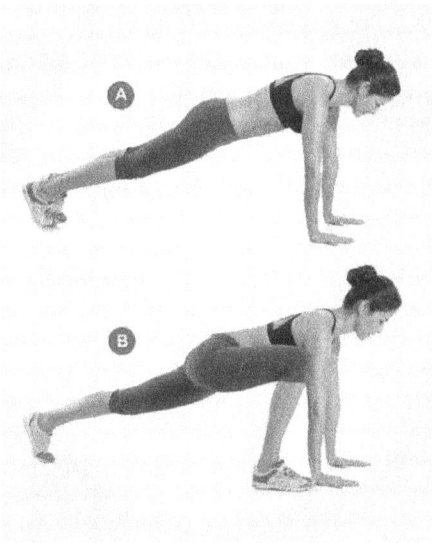

1. Lower yourself into a plank position.

2. Bring your right foot up towards the right hand, hold for a second or two and then return to the starting position. Repeat on the other side. Do this exercise as many times as you can in 50 seconds.

3. Rest by walking in place for 10 seconds.

Part 5: Wiper Waist Whittler

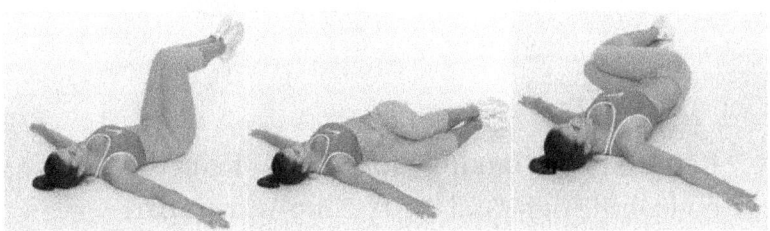

1. Lie on your back with your knees bent.

2. Lower your left knee in a slow and controlled movement until it is at a 45-degree angle to the floor. Make sure that your stomach is pulled in. Repeat on the other side.

3. Do this exercise as many times as you can in 50 seconds.

4. Rest by walking in place for 10 seconds.

The 7-Minute Workout

Tones: The chest, bottom, legs, thighs, arms, abs and waist.
RPE: 5 to 7

Part 1: Walkout Press

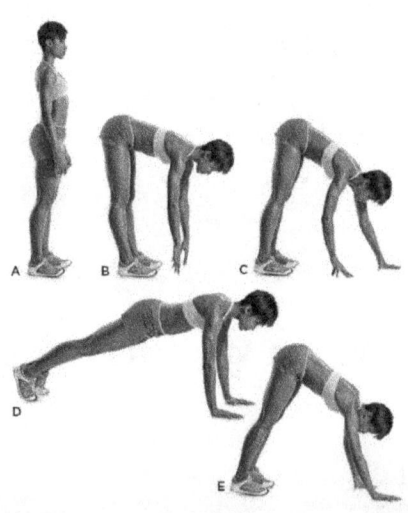

1. Be sure to be standing up straight. Keep the knees loose and a little bent and the feet hip-width apart.

2. Pull in your stomach and begin bending forward until you are touching the floor.

3. Lower yourself into a plank position and then do a single pushup.

4. Reverse the process by walking your hands back up your legs until you are at the starting position. Do this exercise as many times as you can in 50 seconds.

5. Rest by walking in place for 10 seconds.

Part 2: Lunge and Kick

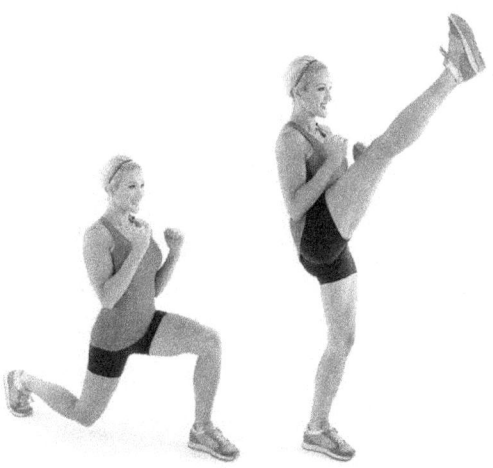

1. Lower yourself into a deep lunge and put your hands on your hips.

2. Straighten up, kick your left leg up and raise your arms until they are in line with your shoulders.

3. Lower yourself back into the starting position. Repeat on the same side for 25 seconds and then switch legs. Repeat on the other sides for 25 seconds.

4. Rest by walking in place for 10 seconds.

Part 3: Jump Up

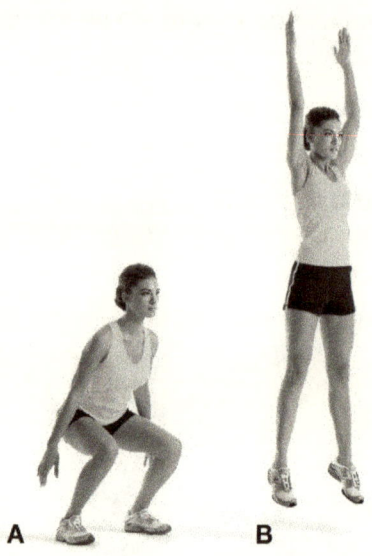

1. Lower yourself to the floor, facing down with your arms reaching out above the head.

2. Get up as fast as you are able and do a high jump.

3. Lower yourself back into the position on the floor. Do this exercise as many times as you can in 50 seconds.

4. Rest by walking in place for 10 seconds.

Part 4: Hop

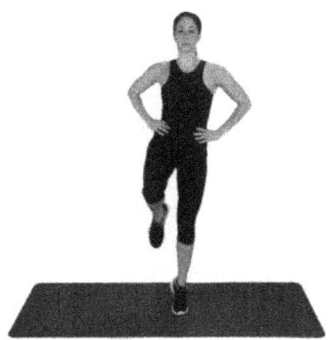

1. Hop up and down on one leg for the full 25 seconds.

2. Change legs and repeat with the other leg for 25 seconds. It is important to keep the core strong by standing up straight and pulling in your stomach.

3. Rest by walking in place for 10 seconds.

Part 5: V Crunch

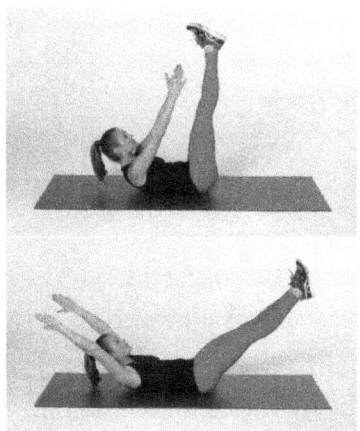

1. Put your hands and your feet flat on the floor.

2. Extend your left leg out behind you and lift it as high as you can.

3. Hold for a second before bringing your left knees into your chest. Do this exercise as many times as you can in 25 seconds before switching over to the other side.

4. Rest by walking in place for 10 seconds.

Part 6: Shaping Your Abs

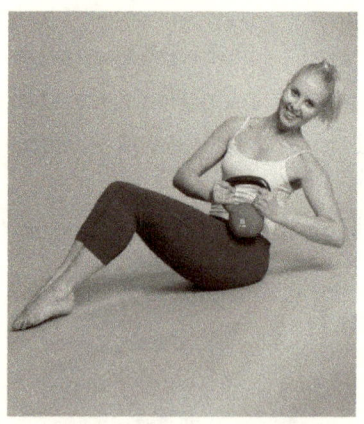

1. Sit flat on the floor.

2. Bend the knees and keep your feet flat.

3. Reach around with your right hand, twisting your body to the left as you go. If you want to intensify this exercise, lean back a little. Repeat on the other side. Do this exercise as many times as you can in 50 seconds.

4. Rest by walking in place for 10 seconds.

Part 7: Facedown Knee to Chest

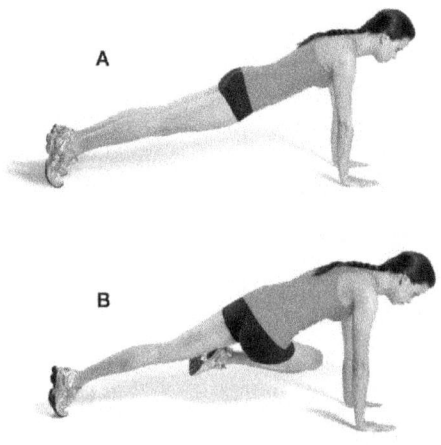

1. Lower yourself to the floor and place your hands just in front of the shoulders. (As if you were going to do a pushup).

2. Bring your left knee up to your chest. Repeat with the right knee. Do this exercise as many times as you can in 50 seconds.

3. Rest by walking in place for 10 seconds.

HIIT For Beginners

Tones: Arms, abs, bottom and legs
RPE: 5 to 6

This is a little easier for beginners or those who haven't done much in the way of exercise in the past few years.

Part 1: Walk It Baby

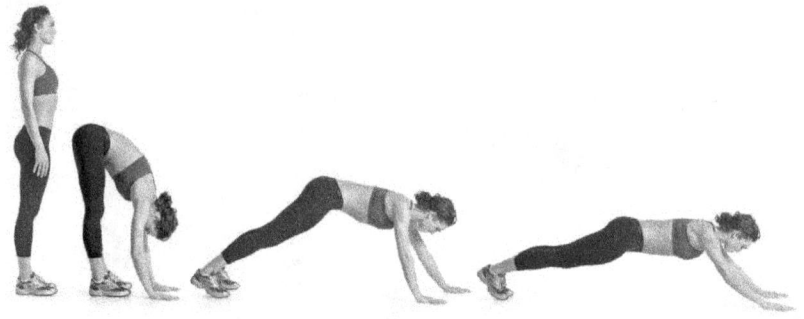

1. Start by standing up nice and straight with your knees loose and a little bent and your feet hip-width apart. Pull in your stomach.

2. Walk your hands along the front of the legs until you are touching the floor. Continue walking your hands out in front of you until you are in a plank position.

3. Hold for two seconds, paying attention to keeping the stomach pulled in and the back straight.

4. Reverse the movement by walking your hands back up until you are back in the starting position. Do this exercise as many times as you can in 40 seconds.

5. Rest by walking in place for 20 seconds.

Part 2: Kick it Out Move

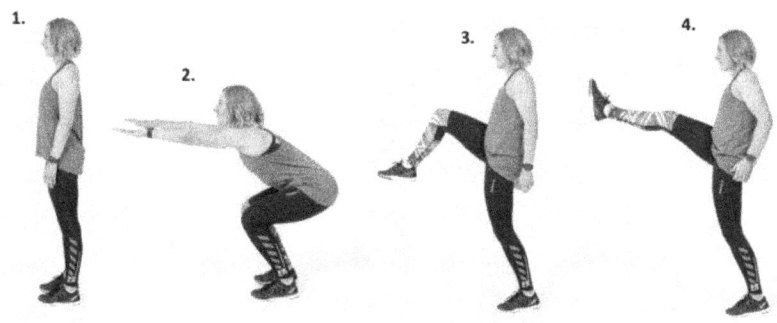

1. Lower yourself into a squatting position. Your knees should always stay behind your toes.

2. Raise your arms out to the front and keep them there for a couple of seconds.

3. Stand up as quickly as you can and kick your left leg out to the front.

4. Bring both arms behind your back, with the palms facing out. Return to the squatting position and repeat on the other side. Do this exercise as many times as you can in 40 seconds.

5. Rest by walking in place for 20 seconds.

Part 3: 180-Degree Turn

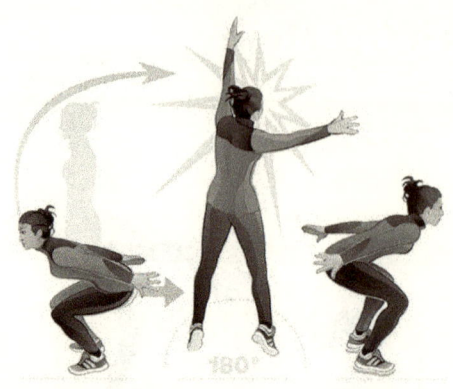

1. Be sure to stand up straight with your stomach pulled in.

2. Jump and twist yourself around so that you land facing the wall opposite to the one you were facing originally. Don't worry about trying to jump very high.

3. Stay in position for a second or two and then jump again so that you are facing the same wall you started to looking at. Do this exercise as many times as you can in 40 seconds.

4. Rest by walking in place for 20 seconds.

Part 4: Traveling Lunge

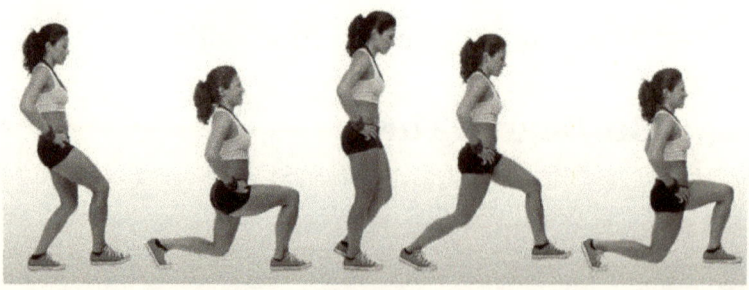

1. Be sure to stand up straight with your stomach pulled in.

2. Step forward with your left foot and lower yourself into a lunge.

3. Put your hands on your hips and hold for a couple of seconds.

4. Take another step forward using the other foot and go into a lunge. Do this the whole way as you move over the length of the room. Do this exercise as many times as you can in 40 seconds.

5. Rest by walking in place for 20 seconds.

HIIT for the Park Bench

Tones: The chest, thighs, legs, bottom, back, waist and abs.
RPE: 5 to 7.

If you cannot find a park bench, any bench that has no back will work. Just make sure that it is sturdy and will support your weight if you are leaning on it.

Part 1: Bunny Hops

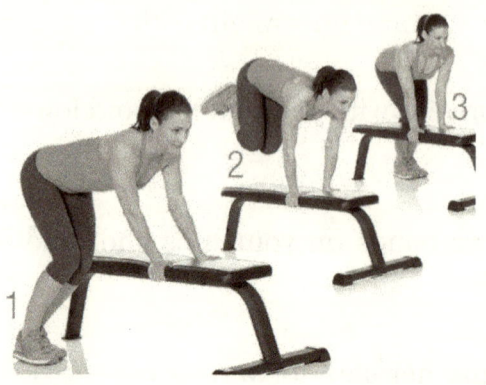

1. Stand to the left of the bench and grasp it firmly.

2. Loosen up your knees and jump up as high as you can so that you land on the opposite side of the bench.

3. Without pausing, jump back. Repeat 40 times.

4. Rest by walking in place for 10 seconds.

Part 2: Bench Push-Up

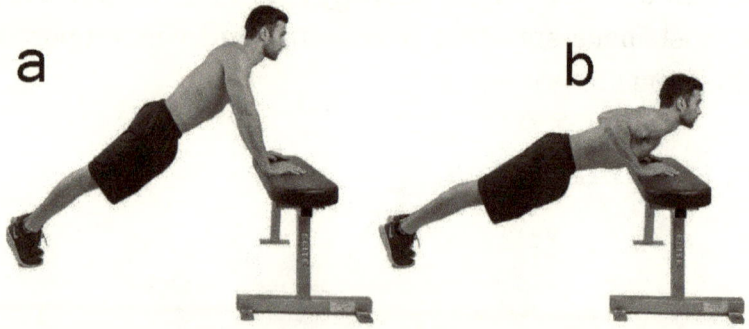

1. Place yourself in position as you would for a push-up, with your feet on the floor and arms on the bench.

2. Pull in your stomach and make sure that the rest of your body forms a straight line.

3. Do a total of 25 pushups.

4. Rest by walking in place for 10 seconds.

Part 3: Step It Up

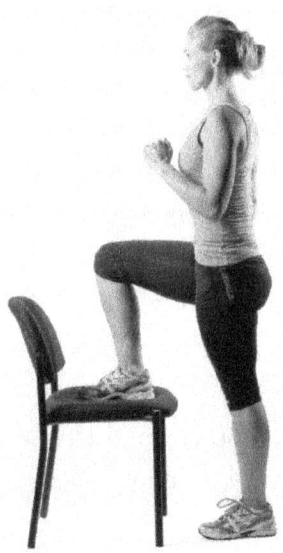

1. Face the bench and then step up onto it, leading with your left leg.

2. Repeat this twenty times and then change over to the right leg. If you want to increase the intensity, you can also add a little jump in between each step up.

3. Rest by walking in place for 10 seconds.

Part 4: Arm Dips

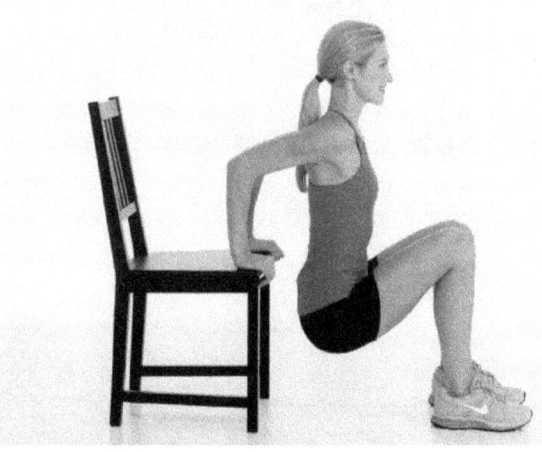

1. Position yourself on the very edge of the bench seat.

2. Keep your arms at your sides, ensuring that they are spaced a little more than shoulder-width apart.

3. Push yourself off the edge of the seat and lower yourself towards the ground a little.

4. Push yourself back up to the starting position. Repeat for a total of 20 times. If this is becoming too easy for you, try walking your feet out before the dip. The further they are from the bench, the harder this exercise will become.

5. Rest by walking in place for 10 seconds.

Part 5: Step-Up Knee Lift

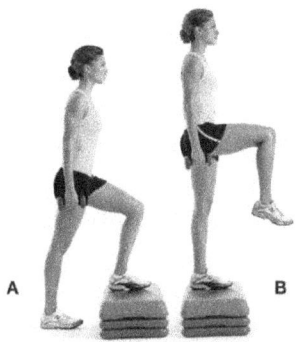

1. Stand to the left of the park bench.

2. Step up onto the bench with your right leg. At the same time, raise your left knee and your left arm.

3. Stay in this position for a second and then return to the starting position. Do a total of 20 repetitions on each side of the body.

4. Rest by walking in place for 10 seconds.

Part 6: V-Crunch II

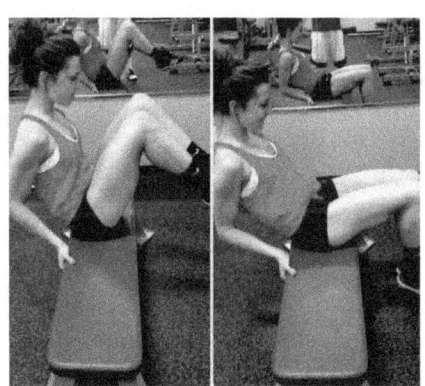

This is quite a bit different to the V-Crunch we saw previously.

1. Sit in the middle of the bench so that you have its full support.

2. Place your hands behind your back and grasp the bench firmly.

3. Lean back a little and make sure that your stomach muscles are pulled in.

4. Bend your legs and then lift them in a slow controlled movement. As you lift your legs higher, lean back a little more.

5. Hold in place for about a second. Repeat for a total of 20 times.

6. Rest by walking in place for 40 seconds.

7. Repeat the entire routine.

Home Workout

Tones: The arms, thigh, bottom, legs and abs.
RPE: 5 to 7

Part 1: T Lunge

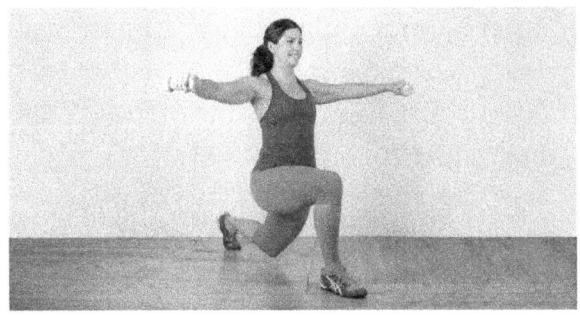

1. Lower yourself into a lunging position and extend your arms out to the sides. Your arms should line up with the shoulders and your palms should face the ground.

2. Push yourself back up into the starting position without putting your arms down.

3. Stand for a second and then lunge using the other leg. Repeat fifty times in total.

4. Rest by walking in place for 10 seconds.

Part 2: Side Drops

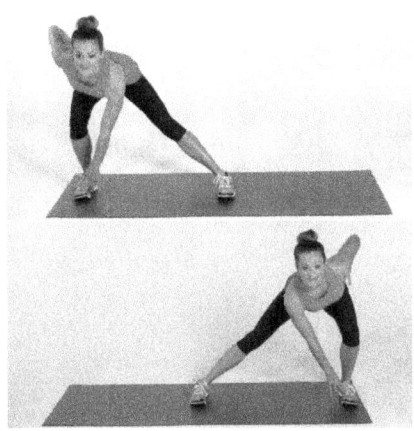

1. Stand up nice and straight, with your stomach pulled in.

2. Extend your arms out in front of you. They should be kept at shoulder height.

3. Lunge to the side using your left leg and reach over so that you can touch the ground using your right hand. Stay in this position for a second before returning back to the starting position.

4. Repeat the exercise using the opposite leg and arm. Complete a total of 50 reps of this exercise.

5. Rest by walking in place for 10 seconds.

Part 3: Plank Leg Cross

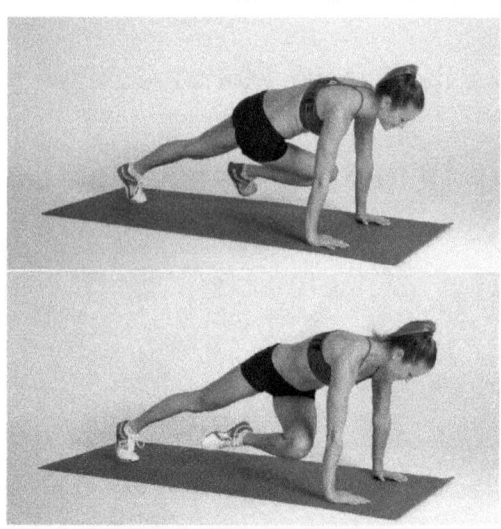

1. Start by lowering yourself into a plank position. Make sure that your stomach muscles are pulled in tightly.

2. With a controlled motion, pass your left leg under the right side of your body. Hold for a second and then return to the starting position.

3. Pass your right leg under the left side of your body. Hold for a second and then return to the starting position. Repeat for a total of 40 reps.

4. Rest by walking in place for 10 seconds.

Part 4: Touch the Floor Drop

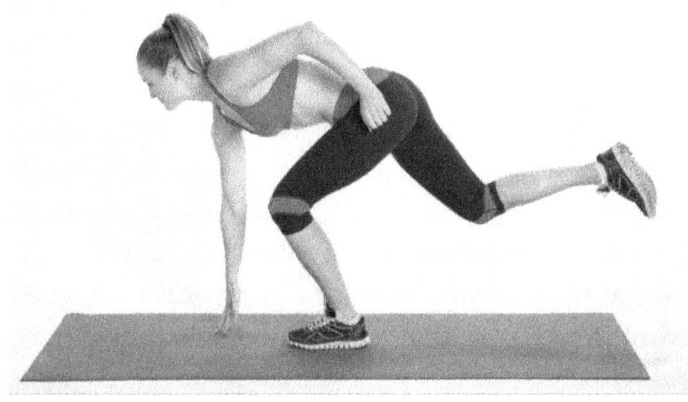

1. Stand up nice and straight with your stomach pulled in.

2. Extend your right leg out a little behind you. Lift your arms until they are in line with your shoulders.

3. Bend forward, keeping your right leg extended out behind you and touch the floor with your fingers. Hold for a minute. Your head should be kept above the level of your heart for this exercise. Repeat for a total of 40 reps.

4. Rest by walking in place for 10 seconds.

Part 5: Ab Leg Lift Toner

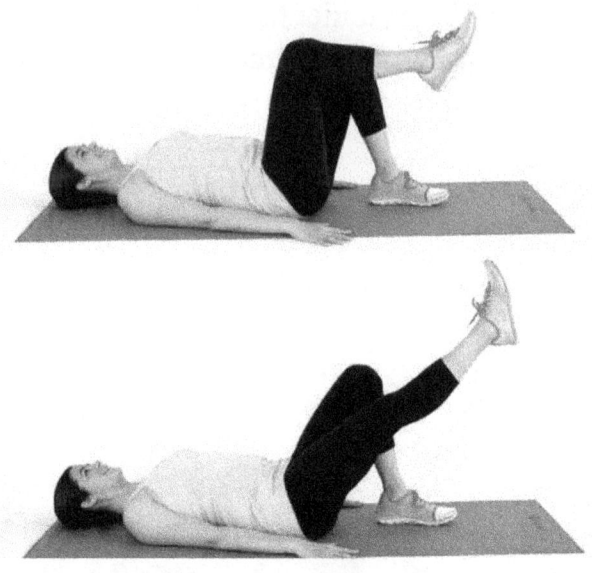

1. In a seated position with your arms bent and fingertips by the sides of your head, extend your left leg out to the front. Make sure that your stomach is pulled in tightly.

2. Bend the knee of the left leg so that the foot touches the floor.

3. Extend your right leg in the same manner. Bend the knee so that the foot touches the floor. If you feel that this is too easy, make it harder by leaning backwards. Repeat for a total of 40 reps.

4. Rest by walking in place for 10 seconds.

Part 6: High and Low Move

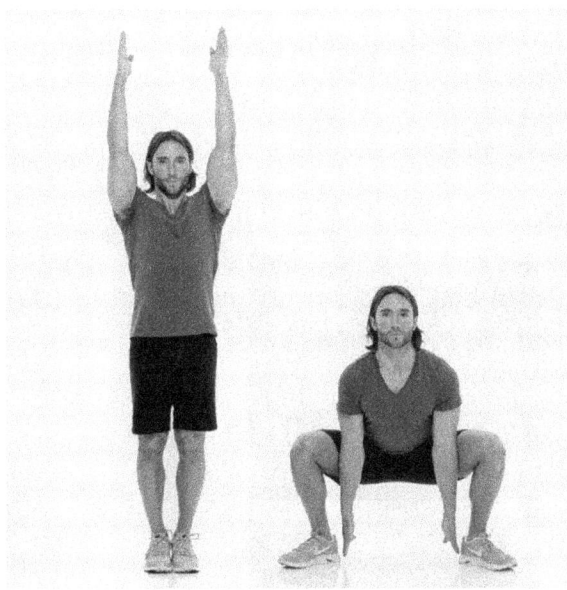

1. Raise yourself up so you are standing on tiptoes. Extend your arms over your head.

2. Lower yourself into a deep squat and then touch the floor using your right hand.

3. Stay in this position for a second and then return to the starting position. Repeat on the other side of the body. Repeat for a total of 40 reps.

4. Rest by walking in place for 40 seconds.

5. Do a second round of the complete workout but this time decrease the number of reps by half.

The Strengthening HIIT Program

Tones: The calves, bottom, abs, legs, chest, back, shoulders and biceps.
RPE: 5.5 to 7.5

This workout is all about building upper-body strength and increasing stamina and speed. The push-ups help to develop the arms, chest, and abs, and the plyometric jumps help increase stamina, speed, and endurance.

Part 1: Power Side-To-Side Squat

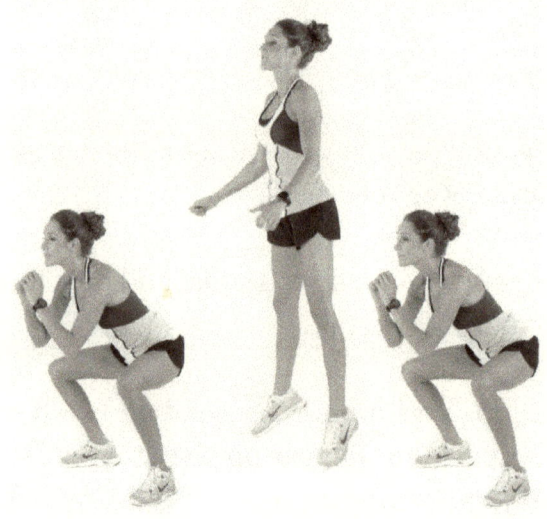

1. Start in a deep squat position with arms in front of you.

2. Jump up high to the right and land in a deep squat.

3. Hold and then jump up high to the left, landing again in a deep squat. Repeat for a total of 40 seconds.

4. Rest by walking in place for 10 seconds.

Part 2: Push-Up

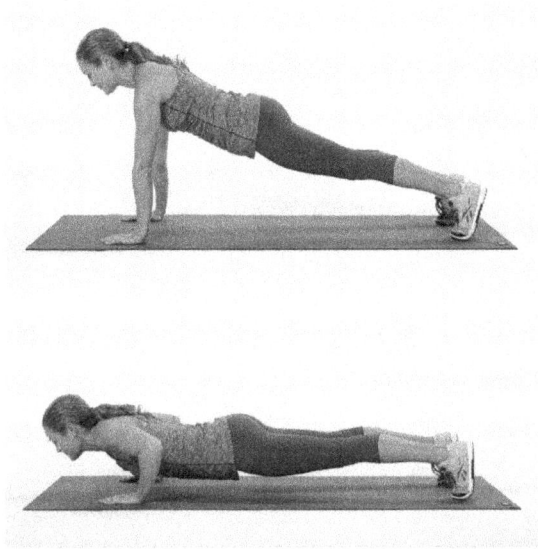

1. Starting in a full push-up position, slowly lower your chest to the ground, keeping tummy muscles pulled in. Aim for 50 repetitions. If you need to rest, that's fine.

2. Rest for 10 seconds.

3. Come into a kneeling position to give the upper body a little rest. Then finish the remaining repetitions.

Part 3: Knee Tuck Jump

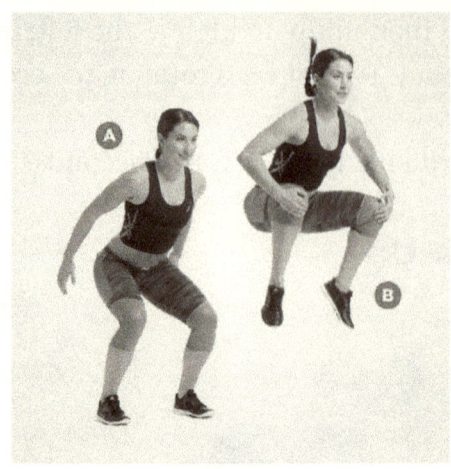

1. Stand with good posture and your knees slightly bent.

2. Jump up high and try to bring your knees into your stomach and place hands on the knees. Repeat for a total of 40 seconds.

3. Rest by walking in place for 10 seconds.

Part 4: Push-Ups

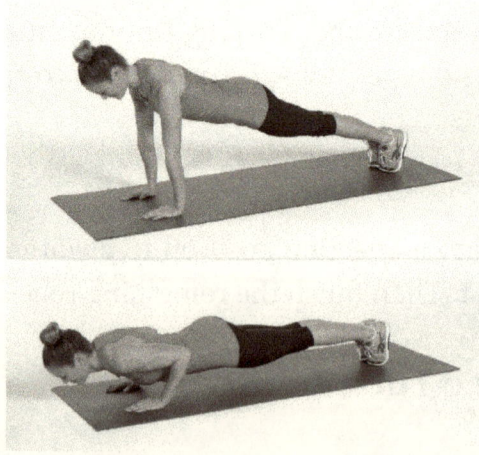

1. Starting in a full push-up position, slowly lower your chest to the ground, keeping tummy muscles pulled in. Aim for 40 repetitions. If you need to rest, that's fine. Rest for 10 seconds.

2. Come into a kneeling position to give the upper body a little rest. Then finish the remaining repetitions.

3. Rest by walking in place for 10 seconds.

Part 5: Left Leg Hop

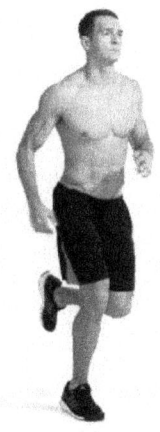

1. Hop on your left leg, keeping your upper body straight and landing softly. Repeat for a total of 40 seconds.

2. Rest by walking in place for 10 seconds.

Part 6: Push-Ups

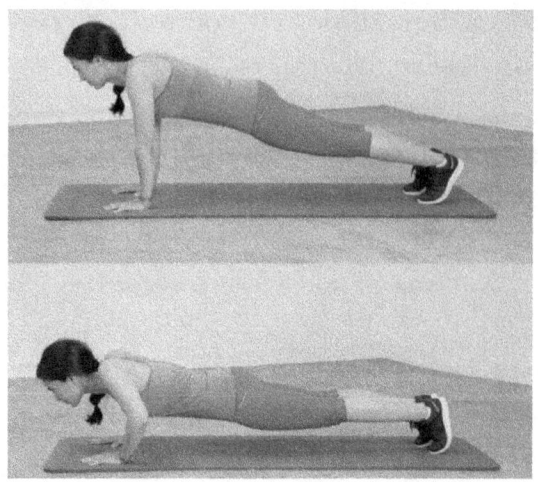

1. Starting in a full push-up position, slowly lower your chest to the ground, keeping tummy muscles pulled in. Aim for 30 repetitions. If you need to rest, that's fine. Rest for 10 seconds.

2. Come into a kneeling position to give the upper body a little rest. Then finish the remaining repetitions.

3. Rest by walking in place for 10 seconds.

Part 7: Right Leg Hop

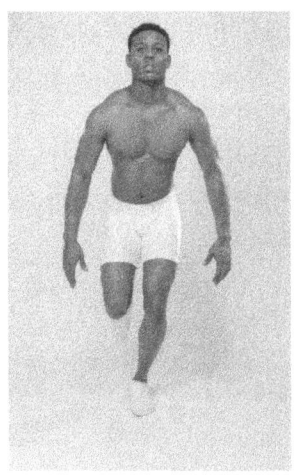

1. Hop on your right leg, keeping your upper body straight and landing softly. Repeat for a total of 40 seconds.

2. Rest by walking in place for 10 seconds.

Part 8: Push-Ups

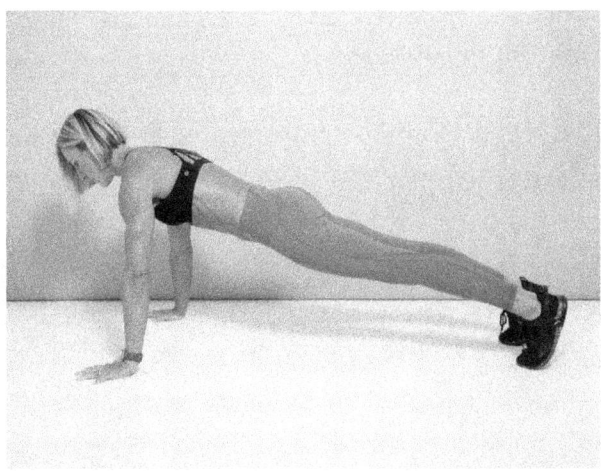

1. Starting in a full push-up position, slowly lower your chest to the ground, keeping tummy muscles pulled in.

Aim for 30 repetitions. If you need to rest, that's fine. Rest for 10 seconds.

2. Come into a kneeling position to give the upper body a little rest. Then finish the remaining repetitions.

3. Rest by walking in place for 10 seconds.

Belly Buster Workout

Tones: Bottom, legs, core, waist and abs
RPE: 5 to 7

This workout consists of three high fat-burning moves that help to strip off abdominal fat.

Each exercise is mixed with an isolated toning abdominal move. You get to engage all three planes of movement, so not only do you get those flat abs, but you also get to draw in those waist muscles at the same time.

Before you start, do your warm-up, and between each round, drink some water. At the end of the workout complete the full cool-down.

Part 1: Star Jump

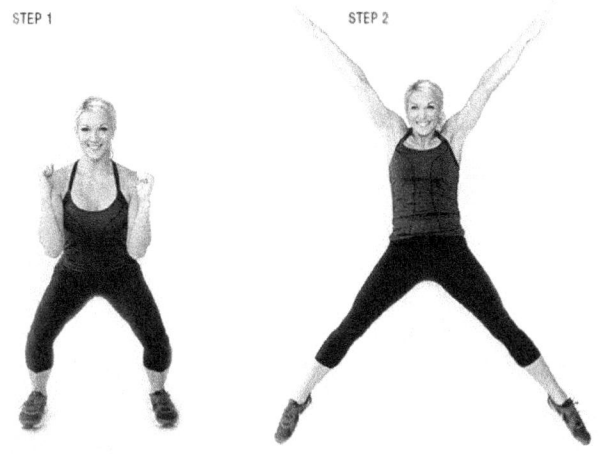

1. Start in a half squat position, with your palms pressed together and tummy muscles pulled in.

2. Jump up as high as you can and lift both your arms directly up. Then land back in the starting position. Repeat for a total of 50 seconds.

3. Rest by walking in place for 10 seconds.

Part 2: V-Kick Abs

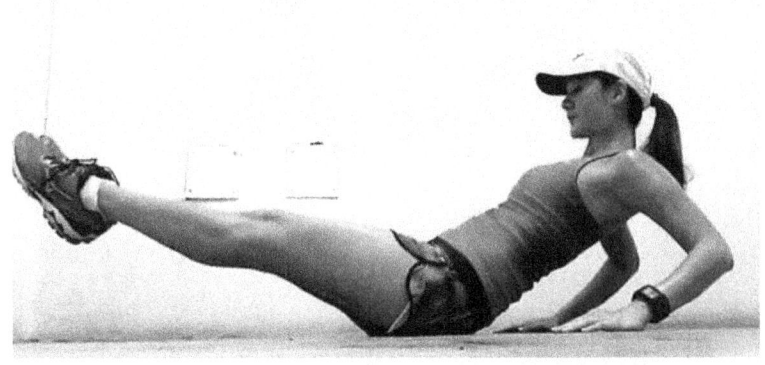

1. Start in a seated position with your knees bent, both feet off the floor, your arms behind you, and your fingers pointing forward.

2. Keep tummy muscles pulled in and slowly bend your elbows, lowering yourself several inches closer to the ground.

3. At the same time extend legs away from you, hold the position, and then draw the legs back in. Perform 20 repetitions slowly. It is very important throughout the exercise that you constantly engage your
4. abdominal muscles; the closer you get to the ground, the harder you work.

5. Rest by walking in place for 10 seconds.

Part 3: Scissor Jump

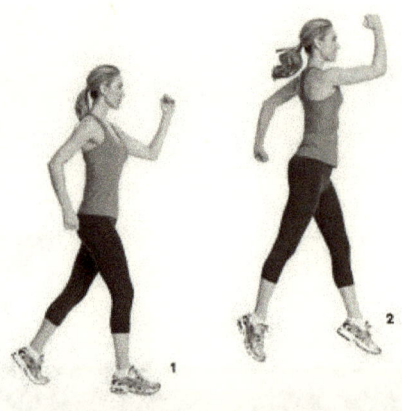

1. Start in an exaggerated march position.

2. Then jump in the air while simultaneously switching the arms and legs. Repeat for a total of 50 seconds.

3. Rest by walking in place for 10 seconds.

Part 4: Reach It Up Abs

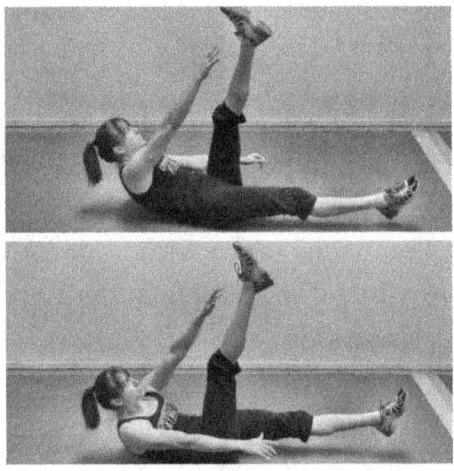

1. Lower yourself to the floor with both legs fully extended and hip-width apart.

2. Place your fingertips on either side of your head and lift your head, and shoulders off the floor.

3. Hold this position and then extend the left arm straight up, trying to touch the right foot.

4. Hold for a second and then change arms, trying to touch the right hand to the left foot. Repeat a total of 40 reps.

5. Rest by walking in place for 10 seconds.

Part 5: Cardio Punch

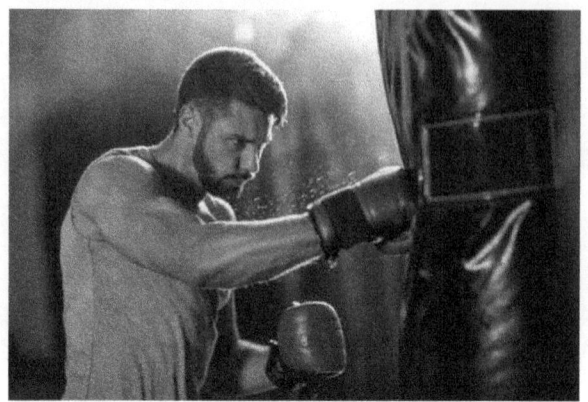

1. Standing in a wide stance with your knees slightly bent and tummy pulled in, punch as hard and as fast as you can from side to side.

2. It is important that you keep the hips still and just focus on the move coming from the upper body. Repeat for a total of 50 seconds.

3. Rest by walking in place for 10 seconds.

Part 6: Plank It

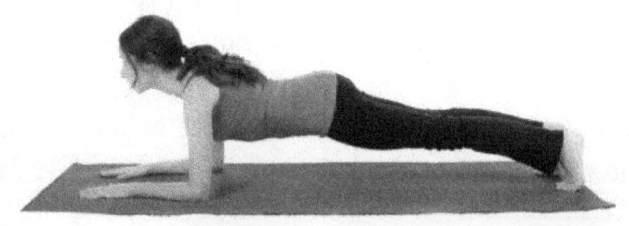

1. Get in a plank position with your toes tucked under and elbows directly under your shoulders.

2. Try to keep your body in a straight line, pulling belly button tight toward the spine. Repeat for a total of 30 seconds.

3. Rest by walking in place for 40 seconds.

4. Now repeat the whole routine two times.

Body Sculpting Blast

Tones: Abs, obliques, shoulders, bottom, legs, triceps, biceps and chest.
RPE: 6 to 7

This workout is tough one and works on stripping off excess body fat. The plyometric moves, done for 40-second bursts, will take you to a level 7.

This is the HIIT part of the workout. You then have 10 seconds of recovery before moving straight on to the next move. These exercises work on building power and strength with moves that will sculpt your arms, chest, and abs, giving you that fit, ripped physique.

Always complete the warm-up and cool-down stretches.

Part 1: Power Side-To-Side Blast

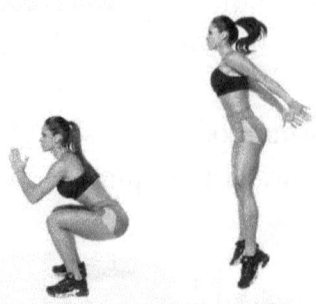

1. Place two dumbbells on the floor several inches apart.

2. Stand by the side of one dumbbell in a deep squat position.

3. Start jumping across them from side to side. Land softly and keep your knees behind the line of your toes. Repeat for a total of 40 seconds.

4. Rest by walking in place for 10 seconds.

Part 2: Iron Man Push-Up

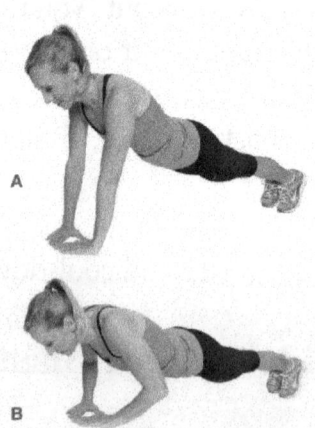

1. In a push-up position, place your fingertips together, forming a diamond shape.

2. Slowly lower your chest to the floor, allowing your elbows to point out to the sides.

3. Then slowly push back up. Keep your tummy muscles pulled in tight. Repeat for a total of 20 reps.

4. Rest by walking in place for 10 seconds.

Part 3: Jumping Lunge

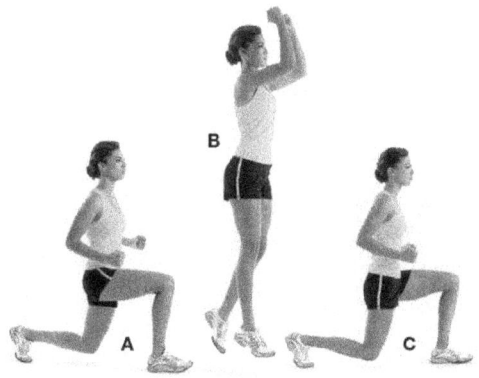

1. Start in a lunge position with the left leg in front.

2. Jump up, switching legs in the air, and land in a lunge position with the right leg in front. Always keep your upper body straight and land softly. Repeat for a total of 40 seconds.

3. Rest by walking in place for 10 seconds.

Part 4: Rock Hard Abs

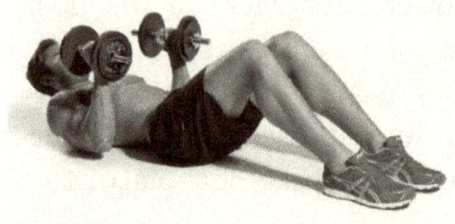

1. Lie supine with knees bent and feet flat on the ground, holding your dumbbells (these should not be heavy) on your chest.

2. Pull in your tummy muscles as you sit up and punch your right arm across your body, hold, and then lower back down.

3. Sit back up and punch the left arm across. Keep tummy muscles pulled in tight as you do this. Repeat for a total of 20 seconds. Rest by walking in place for 10 seconds.

Part 5: Mountain Runners

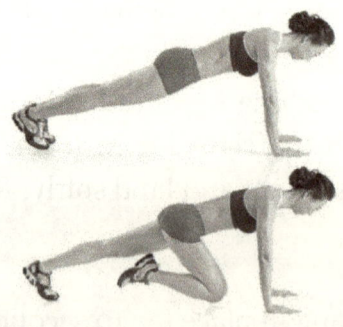

1. Starting in a plank position, bring your right knee in toward your chest, hold, and then place your foot back in a plank position.

2. Now bring your left knee into your chest. Keep your tummy
3. muscles pulled in. Repeat for a total of 40 seconds.

4. Rest by walking in place for 10 seconds.

Part 6: Prisoner Jump Squats

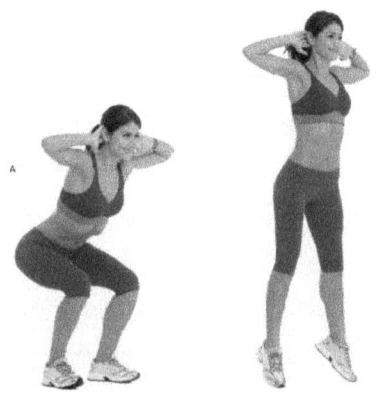

1. Start in a deep squat position with your hands clasped being your head.

2. Jump up high and then land back in the start position. Land softly. Repeat for a total of 40 seconds.

3. Rest by walking in place for 30 seconds.

4. Repeat the whole sequence 4 times in total, allowing for a 30-second rest period between each round.

Fat Burning Faster Workout

Tones: The abs, calves, thighs, hips and bottom
RPE: 5 to 7

This routine consists of just three moves that work your entire lower body. The benefit of this is that some of the biggest calorie-burning muscles are in the legs and bottom, so the more toned these are, then the more calories you burn.

The transitions in each of the exercises also means you get a great cardio workout, so you increase your heart rate.

This is what makes it the ultimate fat burner. Before you start, make sure you have completed your warm-up and stretches.

Part 1: Basketball Side Step

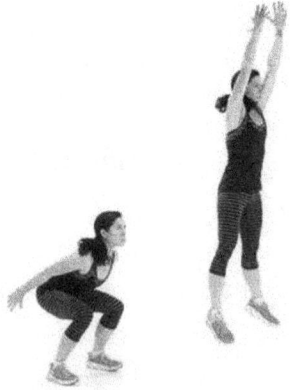

1. Start in a squat position with your arms bent in front.

2. Staying low, take a big, wide step out to your right.

3. Stay in the low squat, and then jump up high as if you are trying to shoot a basketball.

4. Lift the arms at the same time, and then land back into your squat.

5. Step out to the left and repeat. Repeat for a total of 50 seconds.

6. Rest by walking in place for 10 seconds.

Part 2: Jump Squats

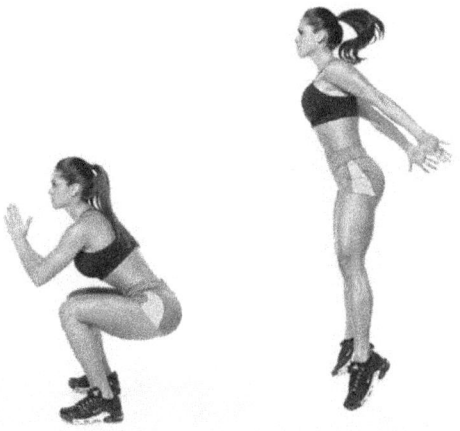

1. Again, start in a low squat; then jump up high.

2. Land back in your low squat, and hold the squat position for 10 seconds. Then jump high again. Repeat for a total of 50 seconds.

3. Rest by walking in place for 10 seconds.

Part 3: Ultimate Leg Toner

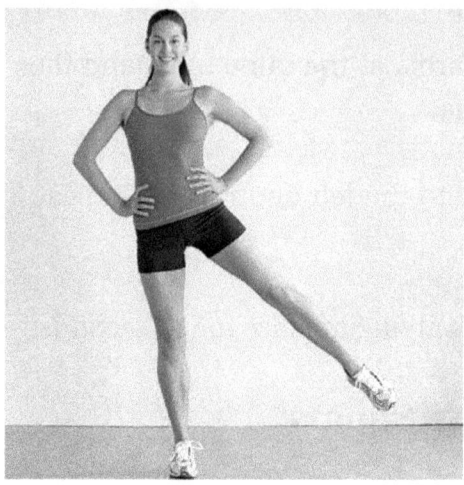

1. Stand with the feet close together and palms together in the center.

2. Slowly lift your left leg out to the side with control. Then lower back to the start position.

3. Now lift the right leg out to the side, trying to lift it as high as you can without twisting your body. Make sure the supporting knee is always slightly bent and keep tummy muscles pulled in throughout. Repeat for a total of 50 seconds.

4. Rest by walking in place for 20 seconds.

5. Repeat the whole routine another two times.

6. At the end finish off with a glass of water and do your cool-down stretches.

HIIT Walking Workout

Tones: The calves, arms, hips, bottom, legs, waist and abs.
RPE: 5 to 7

Walking is one of the most natural exercises we can do, and this low-impact move helps to tone and sculpt you all over.

By adding this HIIT workout, you can burn off excess calories and increase your general fitness.

Walking is a great way to tone your legs, bottom, abs, and arms; plus, if you add any hills to your workout, you will then work those legs and bottom muscles even harder, which is great for seeing results quickly.

15-Minute HIIT Walking Workout

1. 1 minute brisk pace: Level 5

2. 30 second shorter stride but faster pace: Level 6

3. 20 second normal stride but fastest pace: Level 7

4. 10 second gentle walk: Level 4

5. REPEAT 7 TIMES

6. Then finish with 40 star jumps.

Good posture is essential when it comes to these exercises. Always walk up straight, keep your stomach pulled in and walk with your shoulders relaxed.

Running HIIT Workout

Tones: Bottom, legs, core, waist and abs
RPE: 5 to 7

Improve your running endurance and speed with this HIIT workout. The shorter bursts of higher intensity will help to increase your pace and improve your running stamina.

When you get fitter, you can add the 15-minute routine provided next to your running. Use slight inclines as the hills are a great way to build power in the lower body, which ultimately helps with your speed.

The 15-Minute Routine

1. 2 minutes and 30 seconds running at a normal pace: Level 5

2. 20 seconds sprinting as fast as you can: Level 7

3. 10 seconds gentle jogging: Level 5

4. REPEAT 5 TIMES

Running Tip

Breathe through your nose and mouth to make sure you get plenty of oxygen to your muscles while running.

When running at a slower pace, focus on taking deep belly breaths as this will help prevent any side stitches.

The Free Weights HIIT Workout

Tones: The abs, bottom, legs, triceps, chest, obliques, shoulders, and biceps.
RPE: 5 to 7.5

This workout proves that HIIT is not all about cardio! You can get amazing results by doing a mix of cardio and free weights, and the benefit of both these styles of training is that they are both high fat burners.

Mixing them together not only helps build a stronger muscular body
but also helps strip off excess body fat by elevating your resting metabolic rate (the number of calories your body burns).

It stays elevated for hours after your workout.

Before you perform your workout, make sure you complete your warm-up.

For the free weights, I recommend you use a weight that you can lift for at least 8 to 12 repetitions before it feels challenging, so a
good guide is to find the weight that hits that challenge point.

If you feel challenged after a few repetitions, the weight is too heavy, and if you feel you could keep going after 25 repetitions, the weight is too light.

Part 1: High Knees in Place

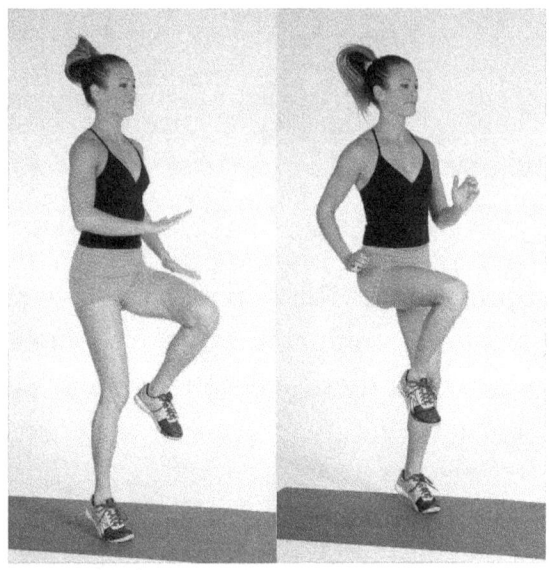

1. Running in place, try to get your knees high, pumping through with your arms.

2. Keep your back straight and land softly. Repeat for a total of 60 seconds.

3. Rest by walking in place for 10 seconds.

Part 2: Alternating Bicep Curls

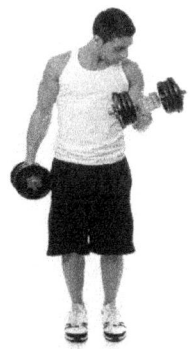

1. Stand straight with your arms bent so both weights are by your chest.

2. Slowly start to lower one weight down toward your hip. You are straightening the arm.

3. Then lift the weight back up and switch arms. Repeat for a total of 20 reps.

4. Rest by walking in place for 10 seconds.

Part 3: High Knees in Place

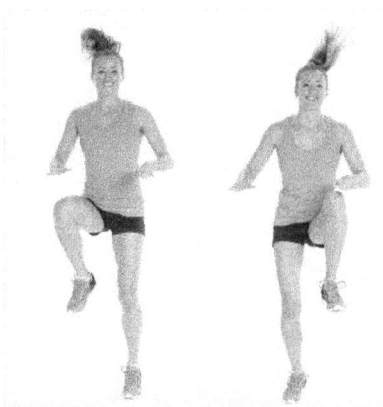

1. Running in place, try to get your knees high, pumping through with your arms.

2. Keep your back straight and land softly. Repeat for a total of 50 seconds.

3. Rest by walking in place for 10 seconds.

Part 4: Weighted Side Bends

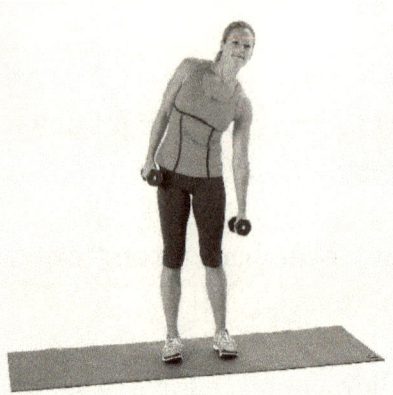

1. Hold your free weights on either side of your body.

2. Slowly bend to one side, lowering the weight toward your knee while bringing the other weight up close to your chest.

3. Hold for a second and then slowly lower back down, alternating from side to side. It is important that you keep your knees soft and your tummy muscles pulled in. Don't lean forward or backward. Repeat for a total of 22 reps.

4. Rest by walking in place for 10 seconds.

Part 5: High Knees in Place

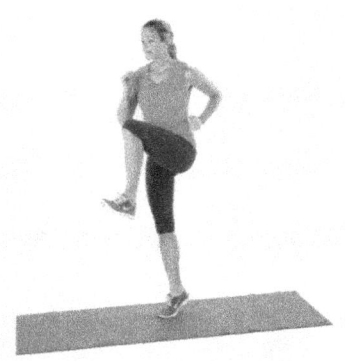

1. Running in place, try to get your knees high, pumping through with your arms.

2. Keep your back straight and land softly. Repeat for a total of 40 seconds.

3. Rest by walking in place for 10 seconds.

Part 6: Weighted Squat

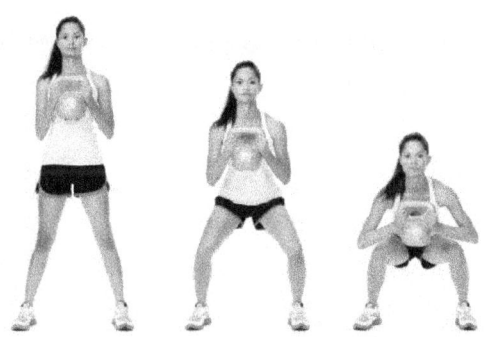

1. Stand straight with good posture and your arms down at your sides, holding onto your free weights.

2. Slowly bend, coming into a squat. Try to get the weights as close to the floor as you can and then push back up. Repeat for a total of 60 reps.

3. Rest by walking in place for 10 seconds.

Part 7: High Knees in Place

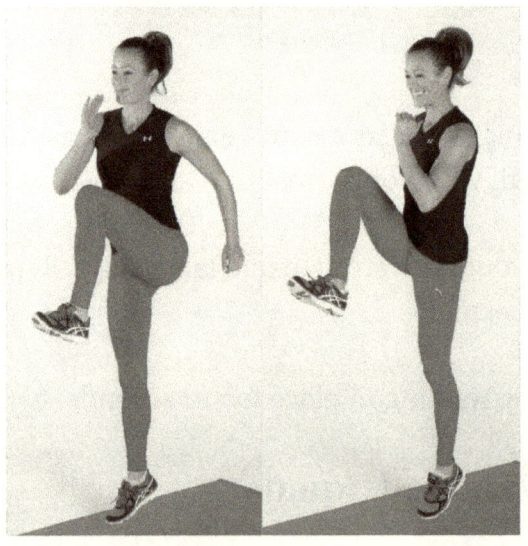

1. Running in place, try to get your knees high, pumping through with your arms.

2. Keep your back straight and land softly. Repeat for a total of 30 seconds.

3. Rest by walking in place for 10 seconds.

Part 8: Free Weight Lunge

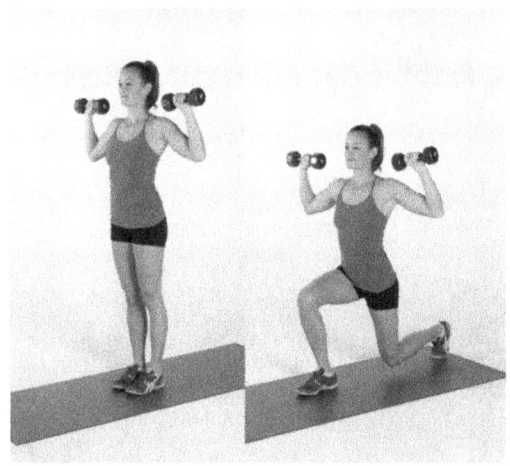

1. Stand with good posture and your arms down by your sides.

2. Now lunge forward on your left leg while at the same time bringing both your arms up to you toward your chest.

3. Hold and then push back off the left foot and come up to standing and straighten the arms.

4. Then lunge with right foot, again performing a biceps curl with the weights. Repeat for a total of 20 reps.

5. Rest by walking in place for 10 seconds.

Others who are considering purchasing this book would love to know what you think. If you could spare a few seconds, they would greatly appreciate reading an honest review from you. Simply visit the page on Amazon.com.

Enjoying this book?

Check out my other best sellers!

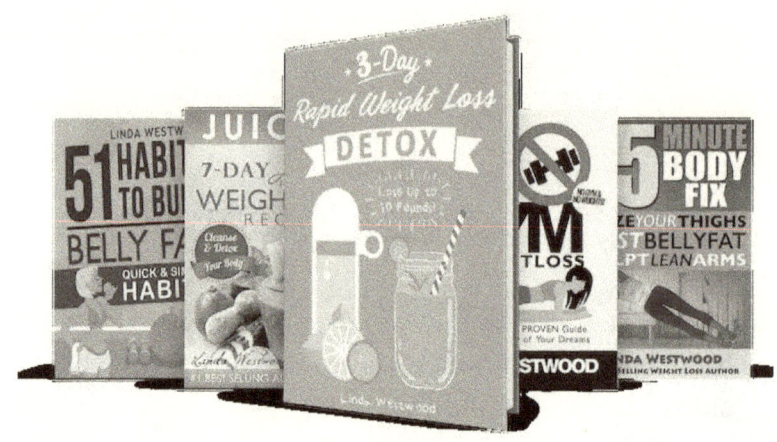

Get your next book on sale here:

TopFitnessAdvice.com/go/books

Chapter 5

The Main Reason You Can't Lose Weight

Believe it or not, your diet is the main reason that you can't lose weight. It doesn't matter how much you exercise, if you are not feeding your body the nutrients it needs, it is never going to be completely healthy.

A healthy diet should consist of a wide variety of foods. This way you ensure your body is getting all the nutrients it needs.

A lot of the fad diets help us to lose weight by making us cut out a whole food group. These diets are never a long-term solution because they are so unbalanced.

Another mistake that people make is to restrict their calories too much. Converse to popular opinion, eating more of the right foods will help you to lose weight.

Calorie counting or restriction is not that helpful when it comes to a long-term solution because it is not sustainable.

Eating should be fun – we need to enjoy our food.

You need a balanced mix of the following:

- **Carbohydrates**

    I can hear those who follow the Atkins diet or Banting gasping in horror. But let's be fair here.

Carbs are not necessarily bad. Unrefined carbs contain healthy fiber that helps us to feel fuller for longer.

The catch here is that the Western diet consists mainly of refined carbs. Carbs where all the goodness is taken out of them.

Complex carbs/ unrefined carbs have a positive effect on the blood sugar and provide a lasting source of energy.

Carbs in their natural state are good. It is when we start messing with them that they become bad.

- **Protein**

Protein is essential if you want a healthy and strong body. If you are implementing an HIIT plan, you need to ensure that you get enough high-quality protein in your diet so that your body can repair itself.

- **Fats**

The virtue of fats has been debated for a long time. Saturated fats were once the scapegoat for all the ills of the world. More recent research is showing that trans-fats are a lot more dangerous, though.

Low-fat diets seem to have a lot to answer for. Whilst eating too much fat can stymy your weight loss efforts, it seems that too little fat can have a similarly deleterious effect.

- **Fiber**

    This is one area that the diet of most Americans is lacking in. Most of us eat only half the amount of fiber that we should.

    Considering how important fiber is to health and well-being, this is something that must be corrected.

- **Essential Fatty Acids**

    Omega 3 is one of the essential fatty acids that is necessary to help fight inflammation and disease. To get enough of it, you need to eat oily fish such as salmon once or twice a week.

    If you do not like to eat fish, you need to take a fish oil supplement to make up the difference.

    If you eat a varied diet containing at least 5-9 portions of fruit and vegetables a day, you will usually be getting enough fiber and basic nutrients.

    Once you adopt a healthier style of eating, you will find that it becomes easier to make the right choices. You will feel better and more energetic naturally and this will motivate you to carry on.

- **The Drug We All Take**

When it comes to following a healthy diet, sugar is one of the most serious impediments. Do you have a sweet tooth?

Even if you don't have a sweet tooth as such, there is a good chance that kicking the sugar habit will be difficult for you.

Take a look at the processed foods in your grocery cupboard. How many can you find that are not sweetened? What about those virtuous low-fat products that you have in there?

When it comes to sugar, low-fat products are often the worst offenders. After all, food without fat is not all that tasty – sugar is added to make up the difference.

And it doesn't end there – sugar is in just about every processed product on the shelves today. It is the drug that all of us take and is the cause of one of the most serious health epidemics that we face.

And don't kid yourself, sugar is a drug. Eating some of the sweet stuff releases the same sort of endorphins that are released when we use cocaine or heroin. And it is just as addictive – the brain starts to crave its next fix.

I believe that sugar is a lot more dangerous than cocaine or heroin. At least when you take those drugs you are aware that they come with serious side effects. And let's face it, you don't come face to face with cocaine or heroin every time you go shopping.

Sugar is a killer. It has been linked to obesity and adult onset diabetes. And its effect on your blood sugar is not where the damage stops – increased levels of blood sugar and insulin lead to increased levels of inflammation. This puts you at risk of developing cardiovascular disease as well. And your body will always crave more sugar, unless you can kick the habit.

Just think back to the last time you had a candy bar or a donut. Were you satisfied with just one? Even if you only managed to have one, that hit will set you up for a craving later in the day. The best way to deal with sugar is to exclude it completely.

When I kicked my sugar habit, I was quite surprised at how quickly I got over the cravings.

Whereas before I had to have a piece of candy or something sweet every afternoon, once I had gotten through the first week without sugar, I no longer craved it at all.

- **Portions Do Matter**

It is believed that average portion sizes have doubled in the last twenty years or so. Just look at popular restaurants and their upsell. You can supersize your meals with very little extra cost.

Increased portion sizes make us feel as though we are getting better value for money. They also mean that we are eating way too much now.

Do yourself a favor, start measuring out the recommended portion sizes. Saying that you need to eat 5-9 servings of fruit and vegetables a day sounds like a lot until you realize that this translates into about 2.5-4.5 cups in total.

As a quick guide, a serving of meat should be no bigger than the size of your hand. A serving of cheese should be no bigger than a matchbox.

Close your fist and you will see what a serving size of fruit or vegetables should look like.

Start taking some time to establish what the proper portion sizes should be. Even if this means measuring them out initially, it will be a good exercise in resetting your portions to prevent overeating.

- **Listen to Your Body**

    The other reason that we are so overweight is that we have forgotten how to listen to our bodies.

    Do you eat when you are hungry or do you eat because it is time to eat? Do you eat when you are bored, depressed, etc?

Learning to differentiate between actual hunger and a conditioned response will be most useful when it comes to implementing your new eating plan.

Once you get used to listening to your body again, you will find that it is a lot easier to lose weight.

- **Water, Water Everywhere**

    The last thing that I want to raise as regards your eating is what you actually drink. In particular, I am referring to the water that you drink.

    Most Americans drink far too little water. And here I mean plain, unflavored water.

    Flavored water is better than nothing but it does have a very high sugar content. (Crazy, isn't it?)

    We all know that sodas are bad for us, but did you know that so-called healthy drinks like fruit juices are just as bad?

    The water taken to make tea and coffee doesn't really count either because these are both diuretics.

    What you need is to drink at least 8 glasses of plain water a day. You can add fruit or herbs if you prefer to change up the taste but this is not really necessary. You will soon adjust to the taste of plain water – I can even distinguish the tastes of different brands and I have my favorite water to drink as well.

I hope you have learned something from this book so far and would greatly appreciate it if you could leave an honest review on Amazon.com.

Chapter 6

Your Fat Blasting Food Plan

Food is about more than just filling a biological need. Choosing good, healthy and tasty food will prevent you from overeating and still leave you feeling satisfied.

What I used to hate about going on diet was that I would always feel that I was missing out on good food. I used to joke that if they made chocolate-flavored lettuce, I would never mind going on diet again.

I am not saying that you can never eat pizza or ice cream again. What would life be without the odd indulgence? What I am saying is that you need to stick to healthy eating at least four out of five times. Essentially that means that having takeout once a week is fine. Having every night of the week is not.

I have set up a sample eating plan for the next week for you. I am going to ask you to be quite strict with yourself this week and that you avoid temptations such as junk food and sugary foods. You will be able reintroduce them again later, but have at least one week where you have a diet that is wholesome.

I guarantee that you will feel so much better after this week that you won't feel as tempted to go back to your old habits.

You will notice that I haven't put down set volumes for you to eat. For this week, I want you to get healthy food. I don't want you to look at this as a diet. I don't want you to feel deprived.

Bear in mind the guidelines I gave in the previous chapter about portion size but don't worry about it too much. Your body will tell you when it is hungry. You may overeat on a meal here or there but you will be amazed at how quickly your body adapts.

What is especially amazing is how well you do after the first three days or so when your body gets over the worst of the cravings for sugar.

I have set this out from Monday to Sunday. You can start on whatever day you like. Switch days if you want to. If a particular portion of the meals laid out do not appeal to you, swap them for something similar.

Monday

- **Breakfast**
    - Oats and Raspberry Breakfast
        - Add some oats, then a bit of full-fat, unsweetened natural yogurt. Add chopped banana and raspberries. You can sprinkle on a few extra seeds and dried fruit to give it that extra crunch.

- **Snack**
    - A small piece of cheese with an apple

- **Lunch**

- Whole-grain pita with salad and hummus

- **Snack**

  - Oatcake topped with half of an avocado

- **Dinner**

  - Stir-fried beef and broccoli with garlic served on brown rice with peas

Tuesday

- **Breakfast**

  - Mashed avocado on whole-grain toast, sprinkled with poppy seeds

- **Snack**

  - Hard-boiled egg with carrot sticks

- **Lunch**

  - Tuna with lima beans, red kidney beans and coriander

- **Snack**

  - A few dates with some cashew nuts

- **Dinner**

- Grilled chicken breast with steamed green beans and mashed sweet potato

Wednesday

- **Breakfast**
  - Bowl of whole-grain cereal topped with some blueberries

- **Snack**
  - Super-Green Smoothie
  - Spinach, apple, celery, pear, and then top with goji berries and chia seeds. Blend with a cup of natural yogurt and enough water to make it smooth.

- **Lunch**
  - Turkey sandwich with grated carrots and hummus

- **Snack**
  - Red pepper sticks with cottage cheese as a dip

- **Dinner**
  - Grilled marinated garlic king prawn kebabs served on lemon-flavored brown rice

Thursday

- **Breakfast**
  - Scrambled eggs with grilled button mushrooms
- **Snack**
  - A few almonds with a couple of dried apricots
- **Lunch**
  - Low-fat tomato soup with half a whole-grain pita
- **Snack**
  - Small low-fat yogurt with added oats and a little honey
- **Dinner**
  - Roasted vegetables served with whole-grain pasta

Friday

- **Breakfast**
  - Warm oatmeal with pear chunks and a sprinkle of cinnamon
- **Snack**

- Oatcake topped with a banana and a few almond flakes

- **Lunch**

    - Avocado with tuna and red pepper and chia seeds

- **Snack**

    - Celery stick and low-fat cream cheese

- **Dinner**

    - Salmon fillet served on quinoa with steamed broccoli

Saturday

- **Breakfast**

    - Poached egg on toast with half of an avocado

- **Snack**

    - Small yogurt with added poppy seeds

- **Lunch**

    - Grated courgette with feta cheese and cherry tomatoes, pumpkin, and pine nut salad

- **Snack**

- Oatcake with half of a mashed avocado

- **Dinner**

    - Grilled chicken breast with a sweet jacket potato and French green beans

Sunday

- **Breakfast**

    - Grilled lean bacon with scrambled eggs

- **Snack**

    - Hot milk drink with a banana

- **Lunch**

    - Whole-grain pita stuffed with rocket, mozzarella, cherry tomatoes, and a few pine nuts

- **Snack**

    - Apple and a small piece of cheese

- **Dinner**

    - Lean beef vegetable stir fry

Don't forget to share your thoughts on this book by leaving a review on Amazon.com. It takes just a few seconds.

Chapter 7

Keeping It Up

Okay, we have now gone through all the basics in terms of what exercise to do and what food to eat. All that is left is how you can maintain your motivation.

We've all been there – at the beginning of a new food/ exercise plan, we are highly motivated and can push through any obstacles.

The problem is that motivation is bound to start flagging as we get more used to the program.

Write Yourself a Get Out of Jail Free Card

By this I mean that you need to accept that there are going to be some really tough times. Times when the last thing that you want to do is drag yourself out of bed. Times when that cheeseburger is calling you and you cannot resist.

Cut yourself some slack. None of us are perfect. You can have the odd slip up. What is more important is that you get back out there the next day and begin again.

So maybe you skip your exercise routine today or you wolf down a big slice of cheesecake. It's not the end of the world. It doesn't even have to be the end of your plan.

If you are too hard on yourself because of the slip-up, you risk spiraling out of control. How many times have you thought, "Well, I have cheated, I might as well just give up" or, "I will start again on Monday".

By treating a slip as a blip in the road rather than a big deal, you make it easier to overcome.

Social Support

There are times when you need a fan club. Post your goals on social media and post your progress as well. This will have a two-fold effect, people will know what you are doing and will be better able to support your efforts.

And people will give you actual support as well – both when you have successes and when you make mistakes.

This also makes you more accountable for your actions. If you tell no-one what you are doing, you are only accountable to yourself.

If, on the other hand, you tell others, you won't want to let them down. (And it's easier to let ourselves down than others.)

Get a New Wardrobe

I can't tell you how many times I put off getting new clothes because I was just going to lose a "bit" more weight.

The downside was that as I was losing the weight, none of my clothes fitted properly. I didn't look as good as I could have been looking and the baggier my clothes got, the less people noticed I was losing weight.

Having someone tell you that you are looking great is a potent motivating force. You don't have to replace everything in your wardrobe but do get yourself a few new outfits that fit your new size.

Have a Slamming Playlist

Take your favorite music and make a playlist that gets your brain and body wanting to move. Choose music that is high energy with a great beat and music that you love.

This helps you to enjoy your workout more and makes it more likely that you will keep it up.

Get Rid of Your Fat Clothes

When I was at my heaviest, I had a range of clothing sizes in my closet. There were the clothes that fit me at the time, the clothes that I could wear if I lost a little weight and the clothes that would motivate me to lose a lot of weight.

When I lost the weight, I hung onto my fat clothes for quite a while. This is not a good thing because it can have quite a demoralizing effect – you are in effect saying that you will put the weight back on again.

Get rid of your fat clothes. If you like, keep one pair of pants so that you can see how far you have come. Ditch everything else.

Make it Easy to Work Out

Is it hard to get to the gym? Then set up a home gym. If you do go to a gym, always have a bag ready for when you go. That way, all you have to do is pick it up and walk out.

Prepare as much as possible ahead of time. That makes it a lot less likely for you to be able to make excuses about not starting getting your daily exercise.

Acknowledge How Far You Have Come

Maybe you haven't reached your target weight yet, maybe you still have a long way to go. Don't lose sight of the victories, even if they might seem small to you now.

Small victories add up pretty quickly and bring your goals that much closer to being achieved.

Celebrate ALL your victories – you deserve to!

Weight Loss is HARD!

Discover How to Make It EASIER to Lose Weight & Keep It OFF Forever (This Is The ONLY Book You NEED to Read)

For this month only, you can get Sarah's best-selling & most popular guide absolutely free – *The #1 Weight Loss Guide*.

Get Your FREE Copy Here:

TopFitnessAdvice.com/Freebie

It's time to stop struggling with your weight loss efforts that don't seem to work.

Discover how you can start seeing real results by next week (without changing much in your life). With this guide, readers were able to significantly improve their weight loss results. So, it's highly recommended that you get this guide, especially while it's free!

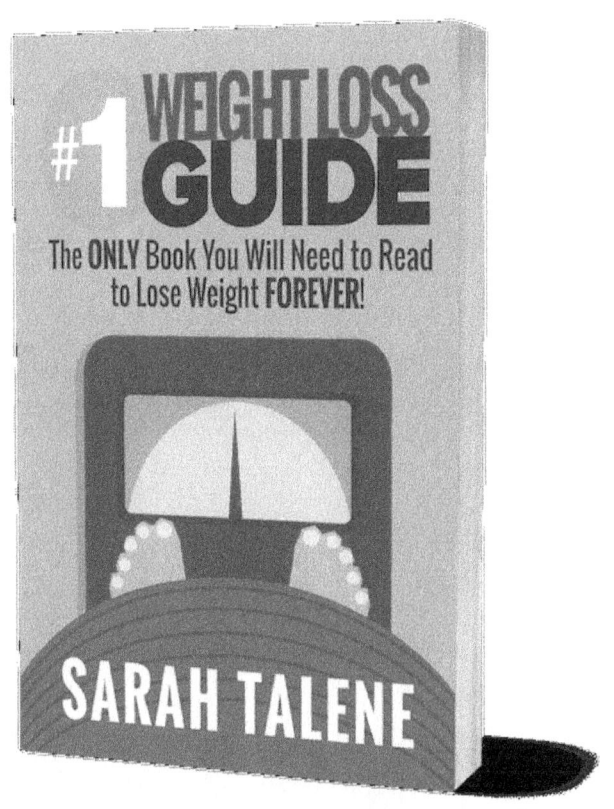

Get Your FREE Copy Here:
TopFitnessAdvice.com/Freebie

Conclusion

We started off by going through why you should choose HIIT over other forms of exercise. We looked at a list of benefits that you might achieve.

My last exercise for you going forward is to make a list of all the benefits you have personally received from this training.

This list is never really going to end – the longer you stick to the program, the more the benefits accumulate. This list should be up somewhere where it is easy to see – I keep mine on the refrigerator. It motivates me every time I look for a snack and it has, time and time again, prevented me from making the wrong food choices.

Now that you have read the whole book and know exactly how the plan works, you are the ideal position to get started creating your dream body.

The combination of high intensity interval training and your new clean way of eating are going to deliver results that you would never have thought possible.

And, most importantly of all, the only obstacle to success here is you. The workouts in this book can be done almost anywhere. For most you don't even need any kind of weights, etc. Each workout is designed to be done quickly.

So now you have no more excuses – it's time to start getting results!

Enjoying this book?

Check out my other best sellers!

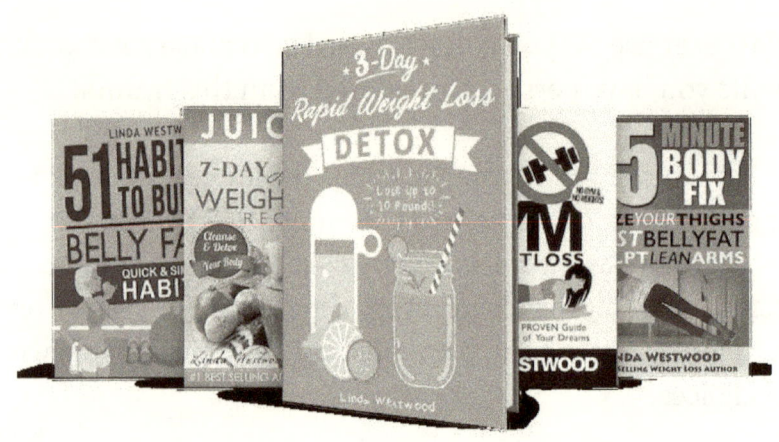

Get your next book on sale here:

TopFitnessAdvice.com/go/books

Final Words

I would like to thank you for purchasing my book and I hope I have been able to help you and educate you on something new.

If you have enjoyed this book and would like to share your positive thoughts, could you please take 30 seconds of your time to go back and give me a review on my Amazon book page.

I greatly appreciate seeing these reviews because it helps me share my hard work.

You can leave me a review on Amazon.com.

Again, thank you and I wish you all the best!

www.ingramcontent.com/pod-product-compliance
Lightning Source LLC
Chambersburg PA
CBHW031157020426
42333CB00013B/715